WHY ARE YOU WEIGHTING?

LIFESUCCESS PUBLISHING, LLC
8900 E Pinnacle Peak Road, Suite D240
Scottsdale, AZ 85255
Telephone: 800.473.7134
Fax: 480.661.1014
E-mail: admin@lifesuccesspublishing.com

ISBN: 978-1-59930-086-3

Cover : Fiona Dempsey & LifeSuccess Publishing
Layout: Fiona Dempsey & LifeSuccess Publishing

COMPANIES, ORGANIZATIONS,
INSTITUTIONS, AND INDUSTRY PUBLICATIONS:
Quantity discounts are available on bulk purchases of this book for
reselling, educational purposes, subscription incentives, gifts,
sponsorship, or fundraising. Special books or book excerpts can also
be created to fit specific needs such as private labeling with your logo
on the cover and a message from a VIP printed inside.
FOR MORE INFORMATION PLEASE CONTACT OUR
SPECIAL SALES DEPARTMENT AT
LIFESUCCESS PUBLISHING.

Printed in Canada

WHY ARE YOU WEIGHTING?

It's NOT the FOOD that's making you FAT!

STACEY GRIEVE

Dedication

To Andrew

You have always believed in me and my abilities, and encouraged me every step of the way! You truly are my inspiration. I love you.

Acknowledgements

Thanks to Deb Elliott for all your support, continued enthusiasm, feedback, and friendship.

Thanks to Karen Vanderzweerde for originally suggesting I put my experiences into book form.

And last, but certainly not least, thanks to my husband Andrew. Your love for me, combined with your constant optimism and patience, were truly catalysts in the creation of this book.

Testimonials

I teach the mindset wealth creation, and Stacey Grieve is effectively teaching the mindset of ideal body weight creation. Read this book, and learn how to get the scales "tipped in your favour forever"!

Bob Proctor,
Bestselling author of *You Were Born Rich*

This book is a MUST for anyone who's ever struggled with their weight and self-image. Stacey Grieve provides revolutionary concepts for changing your body forever. It's the missing ingredient for making your weight loss plan really work - and making the pounds stay off. I've been an emotional eater all my life. This information really explains why emotions trigger eating and what to do about it.

Deb Joy,
Founder, The Primal Bliss

It's not the food that is causing the weight, it is something else entirely. Follow Stacey as she helps you uncover your own hidden reasons for having the extra weight, and she will teach you how to let it go forever!

Clare Tonkin,
author of *Good Vibrations*

This powerful book will help you get to know yourself better, including why you choose to carry around those extra pounds. Yes, weight is a choice, so let this book show you how you can choose to be at your ideal weight permanently.

Matt Thom and Monica Wright,
authors of
World's Fittest Couple Reveal the Secret to a Great Body

The ideas presented here in Why Are You Weighting? *are revolutionary with regards to weight and body image. Let Stacey Grieve show you how to get a grip on your weight and how to learn to love your body, regardless of your size. This book is excellent!*

Debra Ellering-Rosenberg,
author of *Obesity, Not in my House*

Why Are You Weighting?
Table of Contents

Introduction

THIS BOOK IS THE result of years of my own research. Many times, especially in the beginning, I didn't realize I was even doing research; I was just "living my life." It is really only upon looking back over my life that I realize I was doing research, in the form of trying different weight-reduction methods and looking for long-term solutions to keep the weight off.

I literally tried everything I could get my hands on, and nothing, not one thing, worked long-term. I continued to search and search and search, and always seemed to end up in the same place heavier than ever and miserable about it!

Then one day, I started to have a realization. I began to understand that looking outside myself for the answers was not working. Something directed me to begin to look inside myself, and ultimately I found that this was the place where the work really needed to be done. I had discovered that in order to successfully work on my body, I actually had to work on my brain first.

I started to pay attention to the thoughts I was having about myself and about my weight. Wow, was I surprised by what I found!

I discovered that I didn't speak to myself very kindly, and in fact, was harder on myself about my weight than anyone else had ever been (and I had faced a lot of outside cruelty, so this is a big statement).

I found out that I didn't really believe in myself, or even really like myself. And learning this was truly a turning point for me. It began to make sense to me why I abused my body with food — I didn't like me, so what did it matter how I treated myself?

Yet I looked around, and other people seemed to like me, so I started paying attention to what they liked. And the more I paid attention to what other people liked about me, the more aware and sure of my "likeability" I became. And then, the more I liked myself, the better I would treat myself. Not just with regards to weight, but with all aspects of life.

As I got to know myself more thoroughly, and really started to become a friend to myself, I stopped letting other people abuse me, too. I would no longer tolerate fat jokes, abusive remarks, or any other form of put-downs. I began to demand and expect respect. And I got it!

So you can see how much better life became when I began to respect myself. This spilled over into other people respecting me, which literally changed every aspect of my life.

And really, what is self-respect other than "how we think about ourselves? So really what I had done was changed how I thought about myself. But the work was still not fully done.

My weight no longer fluctuated the way it used to; however there were still ups and downs, although much smaller in magnitude.

It's funny how the Universe works! I began a home study business course and, through that, realized that I hadn't really thought of myself as a business-woman. Even though I was doing the work, and getting some results, it wasn't until I started to *see* myself as a business person things began to change professionally for me.

That got me thinking about how I "saw" myself with regard to my weight, and I realized that I had never really changed how I saw myself in my mind's eye. I needed to replace the old "fat" picture with the new me, the slim me, the healthy me. All around our house, I began to remove any and all pictures of me that showed me as being overweight, and replaced them with shots I really liked of myself that were taken when my weight was lower.

The mind always thinks in pictures. Think of your car. What do you see on the screen of your mind? The word C-A-R or a mental picture of your exact vehicle? Same thing for your home. Do you see the word H-O-M-E or do you see the exterior of your house, or perhaps even your favourite room?

Now think of yourself. What do you see on your mental screen? The slim, healthy you, or an overweight version of yourself?

My mental vision of myself used to produce a picture of me at 250 pounds, regardless of what the scale actually said. And so, my mind would operate as the mind of a 250 pound woman, which eventually would lead me back to *being* a 250 pound woman again! It was a nasty, vicious cycle.

It is not easy changing your thoughts; in fact, it may be the hardest thing you've ever done. However, I promise you that it will be worth it! Changing the way I thought has been the single - most effective thing I have ever done with regards to my weight. In fact, it has been the single - most effective thing I have ever done with any aspect of my life! By changing how I thought about work, money, relationships, and fitness, all these areas of my life improved, too!

So, let's get started shall we? You are about to embark on a journey that will finally lead you to where you want to be. I am honoured that you have allowed me to be part of your experience, and that you have chosen me as a mentor.

I won't let you down. *Why Are You Weighting?* was written just for you.

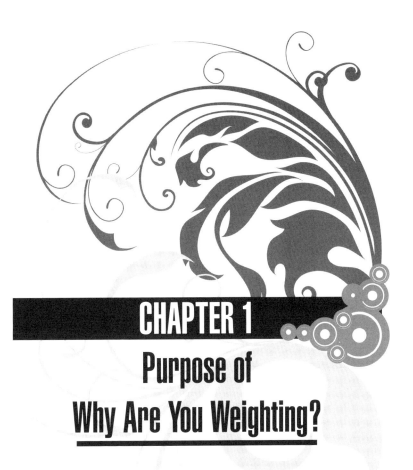

CHAPTER 1
Purpose of
Why Are You Weighting?

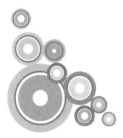

Chapter 1 – Purpose of Why Are You Weighting?

THERE ARE LITERALLY HUNDREDS of plans to help you lose weight. What the world needs now is not another weight-loss formula; we have more than enough of these as it is! Some are good and some are not, and most of these plans, if followed correctly, will result in the scales coming down a notch or two.

But what happens afterwards?

If you are like most people, in spite of your best efforts, it doesn't seem to be long before the numbers on the scale start creeping up again or you notice that your pants are getting a wee bit tighter. Or you look at a photo taken a few months back when you ended your diet, and you can see that you have gained back some of the weight. Or someone who is a bit short on tact says something directly to you. Either way, you notice that your weight is inching up on the scales again. And what goes along with this phenomenon? Invariably, your self-esteem begins to suffer.

And then what happens?

Well, I have found that for most of us, as the numbers on the scale rise, so does our ability to beat ourselves up over it. We start calling ourselves all kinds of names, things like "lazy," or "no-good," or even much harsher like "loser" or "fatso". And then the harder we are on ourselves, the more the desire to eat continues. And this desire can grow and grow and grow until we are basically helpless to control it.

This urge to eat can stem from a desire to distract ourselves from our current thoughts: "I just couldn't keep obsessing about food, so I ate the forbidden fruit." Or we may want to eat as a way to nurture ourselves. "There, there," we may say to ourselves, "I'll just have this one piece of cake, and then I'll feel better." Or maybe we are angry that we can't seem to eat "like everyone else" and so a rebellion of sorts begins – a rebellion against our own bodies and our own hopes for remaining at our healthy weight.

Any one of these scenarios creates a really nasty cycle, which has the end result that we get exactly the opposite of what we originally went looking for. At the onset of our weight loss program, we were looking for a drop on the scales, and a better self-image. What do we get instead. A higher (often higher than ever!) number on the scales, along with a decrease in our self-esteem and self-confidence.

Clearly there is something missing from this formula!

Self-esteem and confidence are two of the biggest allies we have in the "battle of the bulge." When we feel good about ourselves (positive self-esteem) and we are full of self-confidence ("I can do anything!" attitude) we are poised to win, to succeed, to overcome!

And that is exactly what this program is about.

Why Are You Weighting? was designed to help you get the actual results you are looking for. No more yo-yo dieting. No more hiding behind food. No more wondering why you regain the weight. No more beating yourself up. No more food obsessions.

Why Are You Weighting? will teach you to keep the weight off as you increase your self-esteem and your sense of well being. *Why Are You Weighting?* is not another diet plan. As I mentioned earlier, there are already more than enough of those. *Why Are You Weighting?* is a revolutionary new concept in weight-management that is easy, effective, and do-able by everyone, at any stage in the weight management journey.

Whether you are currently at your heaviest, in a mid-range, or even at your lowest weight doesn't matter. However many times you have previously tried to lose weight or keep it off doesn't matter. Whether you are young or old, black or white, rich or poor, it doesn't matter. Whether you are currently on a diet or not doesn't matter. In fact, the only thing that does matter is your desire to reach and/or maintain a healthy body weight. If you have the desire, *Why Are You Weighting?* has the answers. All you have to do is follow what *Why Are You Weighting?* has recommended!

The *Why Are You Weighting?* program can be incorporated into your plan regardless of where you are on your weight loss journey. And the sooner you begin to use these concepts, the sooner you'll get the results you are looking for!

So let's get going!

Chapter 1 Summary

- Most people can lose weight; it is keeping it off that is the real challenge.
- Weight re-gain causes a loss of self-esteem and self-confidence.
- *The Why Are You Weighting?* system works regardless of where you are on the scales.

Be sure to visit www.WhyAreYouWeighting.com and join our website!

_____

_____

_____

_____

_____

_____

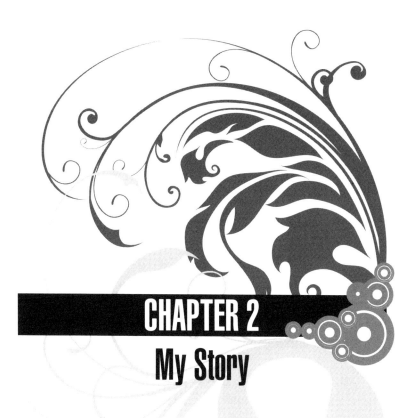

CHAPTER 2
My Story

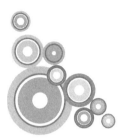

Chapter 2 — My Story

I CAME FROM A FAMILY that ate badly, exercised rarely, and worked too much. Fast food, convenience food, and junk food were staples in my life. Exercise was a word rarely, if ever, spoken around our house. Everyone was working hard, so convenience in the form of quick, easy-to-make meals took priority. "Hamburger Helper," canned spaghetti, and processed lunch meats were the norm.

All this took its toll, and by the time I was six years old, I weighed about 90 pounds. (The average six-year-old weighs about 45 pounds.) Even though I was very heavy for my age, I didn't realize that there was anything really different about me from other children.

I was a gregarious kid, full of curiosity not a shy bone in my body. I remember once when I was about five, one of my friend's mothers commented that I "was certainly a bold child." I didn't know the word "bold" yet, and assumed she meant "bald" and replied, "What are you talking about? I have hair!"

I was also a fairly active child. I loved to swim, and in fact felt more at home in the water than I did on land. I loved being outside playing! And in the winter, I was often found at the ice-skating rink or at the tobogganing hill. I was not a particularly well coordinated child, though, so things like learning to ride a bike, or how to skip "double Dutch" style seemed harder for me than for the other kids. The adults in my life (parents, teachers, etc.) would often tell me that was because of my weight. This was when I started to realize that my weight was something "bad." The looks on the adult's faces said it all.

When I turned 12, my mother was seriously concerned about my weight and eating habits, and shuffled me off to a local weight-reduction group meeting. I learned about "good" food and "bad" food. I figured out that if I ate nothing but cottage cheese and canned pineapple I could lose weight pretty quickly. I learned that a lower number on the scale resulted in praise, while a higher number resulted in shame. Here I learned that my weight was not my own, but something to be publicly scrutinized, debated, and even insulted, often without any thought towards my feelings.

It was during this stage that I realized that a shift in my weight got me attention. I got a lot of positive attention when the weight was going down and a lot of negative attention when the weight was going back up again. Pre-teens and teenagers have various different ways of acting-out to get attention, and I guess this was mine.

This was really the start of my yo-yo dieting stage, which lasted up until my mid 20s, and resulted in my eventually weighing in at just over 300 pounds.

I am sure during those years that I must have lost and then regained at least 300 pounds all told, if not more. In my teens, I was able to drop 50 pounds almost once a year, by only eating one meal a day for months on end. Only, of course, to gain it all back and more as soon as I stopped dieting! My high school yearbook pictures varied wildly from year to year. Some years I am smiling and svelte, and other years I am fat and frowning.

I didn't even go to my high school graduation or prom because I was in a fat-phase then, and just wanted to hide. As all the other girls talked on and on about their dresses, I was miserable, because there wasn't a prom dress in the city that would have covered my girth. My only options were "grandmotherly" dress styles, which would have been even more embarrassing to show up in. So I just didn't go. I don't recall exactly, but I would guess that I stayed at home that night, eating to make myself feel better!

My self-esteem during my teens fell dramatically. Almost every day, someone felt that it was his or her right to comment on my weight or my body. Sometimes these comments were up-front, and sometimes they were more backhanded. I am not sure which was worse, but either method made me feel worse and worse about myself. I began to feel less like a person, and more like an issue to be debated. There were people who were really, really mean to me...teachers, family, even strangers! I began to feel like there was no where I could hide. Where I had once been gregarious and outgoing, I was now becoming more withdrawn, and liking myself less and less everyday.

And the worse I felt, the more I ate. I ate as a distraction so I didn't have to really notice how bad I felt. I ate as a form of rebellion...I'll show you! I ate because I was bored. I ate for many reasons, and most of them had nothing to do with hunger.

So my weight continued to rise and fall and rise again well into my 20s. I was miserable and frustrated, but other than dieting, I didn't know what else to do. I was desperate! I looked into having my jaw wired shut, which they wouldn't do because I wasn't obese enough. I looked into having my stomach stapled, but again, my obesity wasn't morbid enough, so I was not a candidate. They did tell me to come back again though, after I gained some more weight! I recall yelling at one doctor that that was ridiculous!

So, yo-yoing seemed my only "hope." I once passed out in a movie theatre as a result of being on a long-term, 500-calorie-a-day diet under a *medically supervised diet centre.* What teenager should even be trying to live on 500 calories a day?! I now think that is a form of torture.

At the age of 20, I experienced a number of attacks of serious abdominal pain that eventually landed me in the hospital. After numerous tests, it turned out I had developed gall stones and would have to have my gall-bladder removed. This was the type of surgery that is usually performed on middle-aged people, not 20-year-olds! I didn't find out until many years later that yo-yo dieting can lead to gall bladder disease. (The *medically supervised weight loss centre* never mentioned this to me.) After a week of hospitalization following the gall-bladder removal, the first thing I wanted when I was released was pizza and beer, after a week of eating bland, hospital food. And so I continued, eating badly and never exercising. By this stage I was so big that exercise just didn't seem like an option. It was hard enough moving my 300 - pound body around just with regular day-to-day activities.

Three hundred pounds. Just how fat is that? Well, I am 5'7" tall with a big frame. Three hundred pounds was so fat that I couldn't walk half a block without such lower back pain that I would have to sit for a few minutes to recover. So fat that I had to shop for jeans and casual wear in the large-sized MEN's department. So fat that I was horrified at the thought of wearing a bathing suit. So fat that if I found a pair of pantyhose that fit, I bought the entire stock. So fat that the seatbelts on airplanes wouldn't fit. So fat that the seatbelts in most cars didn't fit. So fat that strangers would make jokes as I walked by. Eventually, so fat that I sewed almost all my own clothes, because I could never find anything that fit. So fat that I was miserable!

And how did I console myself? Through food, of course. "Well, I'm already this fat, what difference does it make if I just keep eating?" So I did. Dinner was routinely a large bag of chips and pop, or I would stop at the Kentucky Fried right across from my home and get the three-piece dinner, with extra fries and gravy. Or I would order a large pizza with pepperoni and bacon and extra cheese, and eat it all.

I was humiliated by myself. I was ashamed of myself. I couldn't stop myself. I hated myself. I weighed 300 pounds! I had very little self-esteem left.

Not exactly a healthy person, in body, mind or spirit. What turned me around? Somehow there was a tiny hole in my self-pity, and in this space I decided that I wanted to have a "normal" life like everyone else. It occurred to me that my likelihood of achieving this goal was pretty slim, because I wasn't! Nothing is when you weigh 300 lbs! So, off I went yet again to another diet meeting, with mixed feelings. On one hand, I was filled with hope that this time would be different. And on the other hand, I was horrified at the thought of having to weigh-in in front of someone! However, I guess I wanted to change so badly that somehow I found the courage and went anyway.

After a few weeks on the program and a few pounds less on the scales, a friend of mine suggested that I join a community centre aerobics class with him. My immediate response was a resounding "NO"; there was no way I was going to be seen in public trying to exercise. That would just be too humiliating! However, he was persistent, so eventually I agreed to go with him. Every Tuesday and Thursday we would trot off to this class, and I would be out of breath and dying before the class even got started. But then a funny thing happened. The more I went, the easier it got. And, I seemed to lose weight faster than when I hadn't been exercising. I hated exercising, but seeing the numbers fall on the scale sure kept me motivated!

I was ashamed of myself. I couldn't stop myself. I hated myself. I weighed 300 pounds!

Eventually, I bought a bicycle, and started traveling that way whenever possible. I kept variations of this routine going, and in less than a year I had lost about 130 pounds. And boy was I feeling good about myself! But, again, as soon as I went off the diet, the weight started to creep back up again. When I had gained back about 50 of those lost pounds, I was terrified. Here I go again, I thought.

I knew I needed help. I asked my physician for a referral to a therapist who dealt in eating disorders. I went to this appointment feeling hope – there must be some mental reason why I doing this to myself. I talked with this therapist for quite a while, and at the end of the session, he told me he had good news and bad news. The good news was that I was actually fairly normal, and the bad news was that he couldn't help me. He showed me that dieting just doesn't work, and in fact, it exacerbates the problem. He explained that deprivation (i.e., dieting) leads to excess when the deprivation is over. So, my pattern of dieting periods followed by excess periods was what I had trained my body to want. The answer, he felt, was in no longer feeling deprived by abandoning dieting altogether. I walked out of his office feeling more panic than I had ever felt in my life. If I couldn't diet to get thin, then what was I supposed to do? I was sure that if I let go of dieting, I would end up weighing more than ever. I walked down the street, tears flowing down my cheeks, feeling completely helpless and lost.

Panic set in for a while, and then once the dust settled, I decided that if this guy was supposed to be an expert, I had better listen to him. So I quit dieting forever.

And this didn't work either!

A year or so later, there I was again, with the scales creeping back up. Now, I will admit that by giving up on dieting, the weight gain did slow down; however, it didn't stop completely, which is what I wanted. When I had gained back about half of the weight I had lost, I stumbled across a book called *"Fat is a Feminist Issue"* by Susie Orbach. This book started me down a completely different path with regards to my weight, with completely different results. By this stage I was in my late 20's, and weighed about 240. I started to pay attention to how my thinking was involved in my weight. Over time I began to recognize that the worse I felt about myself, the more I ate, which made me feel worse, which made me eat more. This was not a sudden AHA! but rather a growing awareness of my actions. Looking back on it now, I wonder why this wasn't obvious to me all along. But it *wasn't* obvious to me, just as your patterns are not obvious to you.

And then once I was aware of my behaviour, I then started to think about why I habitually kept putting myself through this never-ending cycle. And then it dawned on me!

I realized that I must be getting some "benefit" out of what I was doing, even if I didn't recognize what this benefit was. There had to be some reason that I kept allowing myself to regain the weight. So then began the process of discovering what this benefit could be.

Now, your first question is probably something along the lines of, "What type of benefit or reason could there be to a situation of increased weight and decreased self-esteem? Why would anyone chose this method to receive a *"benefit?"*

Let's talk here about what a benefit is for a minute. A benefit is something that offers the receiver something helpful or useful. I began to understand that my weight must actually be "helpful" to me in some way. After all, I kept putting it all back on even after I had gone to great pains to get rid of it, so it must be doing something for me, although at this stage I had no idea what that could possibly be. I began to spend more and more time thinking about this. And now, looking back, I can say that this single revelation was a turning point for me.

Thinking about this subject took me down some very different paths, with some very different results. It took me years of introspection to come up with some of the answers that are now the basis for my weight-maintenance success, and for the *Why Are You Weighting?* program. By leveraging what I have learned, and then applying these lessons to your life, you can shave years off your own personal discovery time, so that you too can begin to enjoy a life without fluctuations in both your weight and your self-esteem.

That is really what the *Why Are You Weighting?* program is all about...helping you figure out all the reasons you have for repeatedly gaining back the weight. It can be a long process of self-discovery without direction, so think of this program as your road map to success. It provides the guideposts along the way to your ideal, easily maintained weight. Because I guarantee you this.....if you haven't been able to get the weight off and keep it off, there is something "programmed" in your subconscious that is continually driving you to gain it all back. And until you discover what that is, and then change the programming, you will be destined to keep repeating the loss-gain cycle over and over again. And we all know that is not a great place to be. This is your life, after all. You deserve to have success in the weight area and with this book, and you'll finally get it!

We'll be looking at this in a lot more detail in the next chapters of *Why Are You Weighting?* It is going to be an exciting time in your life as you uncover what is really going on for you, and then make the necessary adjustments to really get what you want.....life at an ideal weight, permanently!

Chapter 2 Summary

- A background that didn't foster healthy eating or exercise is no excuse.
- Misery over extra weight isn't enough to stop the loss-gain cycle.
- Recognize the need for professional help.
- You can get what you want — life at an ideal weight, permanently.

Be sure to visit our website at www.WhyAreYouWeighting.com and join our Million Pound Club, which is a community of members all working to help each other achieve and maintain their ideal weight.

_____

_____

_____

_____

_____

_____

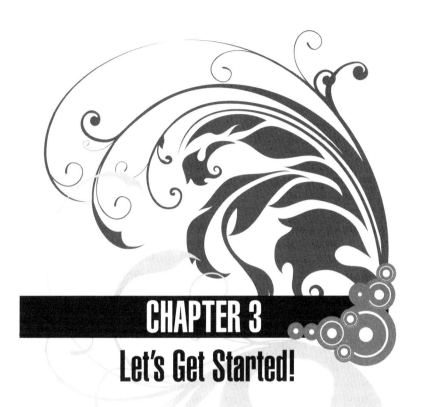

CHAPTER 3
Let's Get Started!

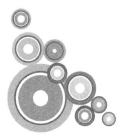

Chapter 3 - Let's Get Started!

FIRST, LET'S LOOK AT the language around weight loss. In fact, let's start with the word "loss" itself. What happens when you lose something? Your brain immediately starts looking to find the item again. Whether it is your keys, your money, or your grocery list, the minute you realize you have lost something, your brain is programmed to find it again. So, from this point forward, we are not going to use the words "lose," "loss," or "lost" with regard to weight. Because if you "lose" weight, your brain is going to want to "find" weight again. I know how silly this seems, and for now, you are just going to have to trust me on this one! So find new ways to talk about what you are doing. You can be reducing your weight, or releasing your weight, or shedding your weight, or finding your ideal weight!

What is language exactly? Let's examine the importance of language. I like this definition: Any system of formalized sounds, signs, symbols, gestures, or the like, used as a means of communicating thought, emotion, etc." Language is a method of communication, and does not have to be verbal. For example, it is often said that "body language" reveals more truth than the spoken word ever does. The written word is also a form of language and communication, and it is often quite different from the spoken version.

We are communicating with ourselves every minute of every day. Some of this communication we have no awareness of, such as the messages that pass back and forth between the brain and the cells. Things like breathing, digestion, and blood flow are all examples of this type of communication.

And then there is communication we are aware of, "Remember to pick up milk on the way home." or "I know I can get this job finished by 5pm if I skip lunch" or "Oh, isn't he handsome!" We know we are having these thoughts or ideas, and generally we act on them if we choose. It is almost like having a conversation in your head.

Then there is a third type of communication we all use, and for the most part, it has become so commonplace that we aren't really aware of it at all, unless we make a point to be. And by far, this can be the most powerful form of communicating with ourselves. And like all types of power, it can be put to good use or bad. (More on that later.) Here I am talking about the constant, ongoing chatter that is present in the backs of all our minds. Occasionally, this chatter gets a bit louder and comes to the front of our minds, and we temporarily become aware that it is happening.

Let's refer to this chatter as our "self-talk." We all have this going on, all our waking hours. There is a constant stream of ideas and comments going on in all our minds all the time.

This is really where we talk to ourselves. Self-talk is also how we express many opinions about ourselves, such as "I'm a great bowler"… "I always get in the wrong line"… "I don't think so-and-so likes me." Self-talk can also appear as "You can do this!" when faced with a challenge, or it can be the exact opposite, like "You'll never do this right you never do anything right." You see, once we start to pay attention to our self-talk, often we'll find we don't speak to ourselves very kindly. In Chapters 4, 5, and 6 we'll look at self-talk, and how to adjust it to be more helpful in assisting you in achieving and maintaining your ideal body weight. In the meantime, whenever you catch yourself saying something less than kind to yourself, notice it, and replace it with a happier thought or idea.

Really be vigilant about noticing your self-talk. Start by just noticing what thoughts are going through your head. Are you being nice, supportive, and forgiving to yourself, or are you thinking things that are berating, belittling, or even abusive? You will be amazed to discover how often something you think about yourself is not really very nice.

We all have thoughts along the lines of "You can't do this" or "Who do you think you are?" which are bad enough, but then sometimes we can even hear a voice in our head that can be really abusive. "You're such a loser!" or "You'll never amount to much" are things most of us would probably never say to another human being; however, we say them to ourselves all the time!

What is important here is that when you do think a negative thought about yourself, be sure to then not berate yourself further by mentally chastising yourself for having had a negative thought in the first place! This is really important! After you realize you've been in a negative self-talk place, catch yourself before the next thought is something like "Oh, I'll never get this right; I am such a loser." Replace that with "I will get the hang of this; it just takes practice."

For now, just notice your thoughts. As you work through *Why Are You Weighting?* we'll be delving further into how to change these thoughts to be more supportive and positive, and then how to use them to really propel you to permanent success. Rome wasn't built in a day, and it is going to take some time to change a life-time of having certain thoughts.

I hope you are reading this book because you are looking to achieve something in your life. And for this, you are to be congratulated! This is a big step, and I am happy we are taking these steps together. And since you want the results this program promises, I must say a word here about the various exercises I suggest along the way. Some of them are going to feel silly, and some even foolish. Anything new feels this way.

> **We'll be delving further into how to change these thoughts to be more supportive and positive.**

Think about the first time you tried to ride a bike, or ice skate, or ski, or ride a horse. They were all strange things once, and they felt strange, and you probably felt strange doing them. However you badly wanted to bike, or skate, or ski or ride, and you put up with these strange feelings until they became more "normal" feeling, because you wanted the outcome, the end result. Well the same thing is going to happen here. You are going to be doing, thinking, and acting in new ways, which is going to require you to step outside of your comfort zone, which is a strange, foreign feeling for all of us.

But one thing to bear in mind....it is by staying in your comfort zone that you get the same results in your life. For instance, stay in your comfort zone professionally, and your career won't advance far. Stay in your comfort zone in relationships, and you'll see that each and every time they only develop to a certain point. Stay in your comfort zone around physical exercise, and your body will continue to look the way it does now.

Staying in your comfort zone really means not being open to learning new ideas, habits, or methods. It means not growing as a person, not developing your full potential in any area of your life. It means you aren't willing to "do what it takes" to get to the point where you are now comfortable again. But just as it was strange the first time you rode a bike, eventually it became second nature. In fact, it becomes so ingrained that we now have a cliché "just like riding a bike," which means that once you have it, you have it and will never forget how again!

Staying in your comfort zone means you are stuck. Whether you are stuck professionally, personally, emotionally, physically, or intellectually, that area of your life is not advancing. In fact, that area of your life is actually dying. Nothing in life ever stands still. Everything is either growing or dying. There is no in-between. You will know this is true if you spend a few minutes thinking about it.

It is only through learning new information and then making new choices and taking new actions based on the new information that we get un-stuck. Notice I said making or acting...these are action verbs. They mean that you have to do something with what you've learned. Just reading this book, and then not taking action on what is recommended, will not get you your desired outcome.

Isn't the definition of insanity "doing the same things over and over again, expecting different results"?

If you keep doing what you have been used to doing (your comfort zone) you are going to get the same results you've always had.

If you step outside of your comfort zone, and do things you may be uncomfortable doing, you will start to get different results, and this is guaranteed! You know this is true in other areas of your life. For instance, if you learn a new skill (which often requires you to be uncomfortable until you have mastered at least the basics) you may be able to apply for a different job, or a better job, or even start your own business. All these opportunities can now present themselves to you because you learned something new.

Or maybe you want to take up a new hobby like skiing. You are definitely going to have to get outside your comfort zone and be willing even to look foolish as you fall down a few (or even a few hundred) times in order to eventually be able to competently ski.

With regard to your weight, if you keep doing what you've always done, you will only get the same end results you've always had. This is guaranteed too!

And you are reading this book because you want to effect a change in your life, so embrace the idea of stepping outside what is usually comfortable for you! Become excited about what you are learning here, and what it can bring to your life, regardless of how foolish or weird you may think some of the suggestions are. It will all prove to be worth it!

Let's just talk about the importance of having the right attitude before we go any further. Have an open attitude about learning. Be enthusiastic about all the new ideas coming your way. Be ready, willing, and able to try new things. Get excited about life and what you are bringing into your life with the *Why Are You Weighting?* concepts.

Speaking of attitude, let's just talk about the importance of having the right attitude before we go any further. The right attitude is the cornerstone to success in any venture, and this one is no exception.

What exactly is attitude anyway? I think of it as the "thoughts about any given subject." We all knew people in school with bad attitudes...those who thought school was dumb, who were disruptive, who picked on others, or who disrespected the teachers and the system. Did any of these people ever do well in school? No, not at all. Some may have made it to the end of high school; however, more often than not, they flunked out, or were asked to leave before they caused others to flunk.

LET'S GET STARTED! **43**

We have all worked with people with bad attitudes. Those who won't do a single extra thing that isn't on their job description. Those who whine long and loud about the boss, or the working conditions, or the pay, or whatever. Those who try to steal credit for other people's ideas. Again, in the long run, how far do you think these people will get in their careers? Not far, I assure you. All because they have a bad attitude around their work.

So what does a bad attitude look like with regards to weight? It can be thoughts of "I can't do this; it's too hard." It could be thoughts of "I don't deserve to be slim" or "I hate exercise." It could be thoughts that "learning about what it takes to remain slim forever is just too much work." Or it could be as simple as "I will always be heavy." Defeatist thinking is really what this is. When you think this way, you are done before you even get started.

William James (1842 – 1910) said it best when he said "The greatest discovery of my generation is that a human can alter his life by altering his attitudes of mind." James also said, "Human beings, by changing the inner attitudes of their minds, can change the outer aspects of of their lives."

Henry Ford (1863 – 1947) knew of the power of attitude when he said, "If you think you can do a thing, or you think you can't do a thing, you're right."

So, as you embark on the *Why Are You Weighting?* program, hold a positive attitude about what you are doing. Be excited about it, not just luke-warm. Have the attitude of "I can do this!" Have the attitude of positive expectation. "If I do what I am told, I will get the results I want!" Realize you deserve to live in a healthy body at an ideal weight.

Success is the result of a good attitude! You literally can do anything if you think you can. And with the *Why Are You Weighting?* program, you will be a success with regards to your ideal weight.

Be sure to also have the right attitude regarding the various exercises that are taught through out the book. Do them as they come up. Don't think, "Oh I'll just keep reading and do them later (or not at all)." Keep the attitude of "I'll do what it takes, and I'll do what Stacey suggests, because I want to get different results."

"With every experience, you alone are painting your own canvas, thought by thought, choice by choice." Those very wise words were spoken by Oprah Winfrey. She also said "The big secret in life is that there is no big secret. Whatever your goal, you can get there if you're willing to work."

This means that you have a choice to do the exercises or not. And each choice will result in different outcomes. Our lives are built by the choices we make, day after day, year after year. Choose to be a success with the *Why Are You Weighting?* concepts by doing what is asked of you...in this case, these exercises are "the work" that Oprah is referring to.

So commit to doing the *Why Are You Weighting?* work. It's that simple!

Now I have mentioned this already, it's worth repeating here again. *Why Are You Weighting?* is not a diet plan! It is meant to accompany your weight-reducing or weight-maintaining efforts, regardless of which plan you are following. And I do believe you must be following some sort of plan, especially when you are starting out. The options out there are endless, with some being much better than others. Here are my thoughts on what a good plan should be all about:

- You should receive the full complement of the required daily nutrients (vitamins, minerals, and good fats). You will learn more about nutrition in a later chapter.
- There should be meat-free meals included a few times a week.
- You should be able to tailor your plan to your lifestyle without too much bother.
- You should have access to support, either in person, via the phone, or via the Internet.
- You should have some access to your favourite foods, even if these are not necessarily "diet" foods.
- You should be encouraged to set goals, and monitor your progress. Accountability is a big factor of success in any endeavour.
- You should be encouraged to reward yourself with non-food rewards.
- You should be reducing your weight at a rate of no more than 2 pounds (1 kilo) per week.
- You should be encouraged to be getting some physical activity daily or at least three times per week.

If your current plan does not follow these guidelines, please look for another plan that does. A good, solid plan will include all of the above. Please visit www.WhyAreYouWeighting.com to learn about our food and exercise plans.

Chapter 3 Summary

- The brain will always try to find that which has been lost. Change "losing weight" to "releasing weight" to help your brain help you.
- Pay attention to how you talk to yourself, and begin to eliminate negative self-talk.
- Attitude is everything! You can change your world with the right attitude!
- You must be following a good, healthy plan, especially when first starting out.

Visit www.WhyAreYouWeighting.com for more tips and insights on what healthy eating and exercise plans look like!

_____

_____

_____

_____

_____

"Because you are in control of your life. Don't ever forget that. You are what you are because of the conscious and subconscious choices you have made."

- Barbara Hall
from "A Summons to New Orleans, 2000"

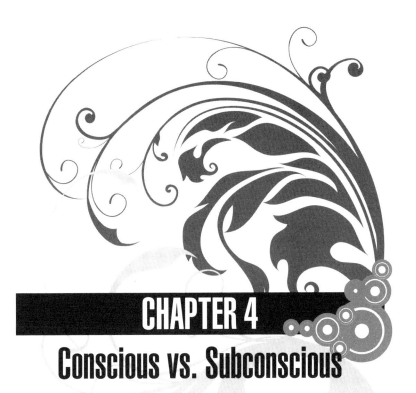

CHAPTER 4
Conscious vs. Subconscious

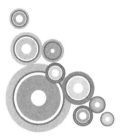

Chapter 4 — Conscious vs. Subconscious

THE HUMAN MIND IS a marvelous piece of machinery! Have you ever thought about it this way? It is unlike anything else on the planet. In fact, the human mind is really what separates us from the animal world. We are the only living creatures that can control our minds and our thoughts, which is different from the animal kingdom. An animal's brain operates by instinct, not by choice. And even the fastest computer on earth doesn't come close to doing what the human mind is capable of!

Now I bet you are thinking, "What is she talking about? I can't do calculations as quickly as a computer, nor can I store (and retrieve) information nearly as efficiently as a computer can." And although you may be right about these two specific tasks there are many things your mind can do that no computer can even come close to!

Your mind has many powers beyond the ability to work with numbers or to store and retrieve information. It is in your mind that the five senses are realized, and here's an example of what I mean. We've all had a fly land on our arm. Now you may think you "feel" the fly land, but in reality what's happening is that a message is relayed to the brain and the real "feeling" happens there. Your brain interprets the message from the nerves in your arm as "there is something on my arm."

It is the same with sight. You may think that you see with your eyes, but in fact, it is your brain that really does the seeing. The part of the eye that receives the image through the lens is called the retina. And we know now that the retina is actually an extension of brain tissue, rather than eye tissue. The various parts of the eye itself manipulate the data coming in through your pupil, but it is your brain that actually interprets it into the function we call seeing.

This same is true for all of our five senses. And beyond our five senses, there are six other abilities that our brains have. Everyone knows about the five senses because these were taught in school, but the six other abilities are equally important! But because these six are less tangible, they are often overlooked. This is a real shame, as these six can be just as important for processing information as the five basic senses. They are memory, intuition, reason, imagination, will, and perception. Since they aren't taught at school, let's look at each of these for a moment before we go on.

We all know what memory is. However, did you know that you can actually train and improve your memory? Your current "memory-ability" has nothing to do with what you are really capable of. In fact, mind experts teach that "memory is perfect" and that we can all have perfect memories if we choose to learn to use our minds differently.

Reason is the ability to think. It is the way the brain looks at the different pieces of information, and forms conclusions, judgments, and inferences based on this information. Reason is also the capacity for logical, analytical, and rational thought, also known as intelligence.

Intuition is often called the "sixth sense" as it too is a way of getting information into the mind. In some ways, it is the opposite of reason, as it is knowing or sensing something without the use of rational processes. In other words, knowing something without really thinking about it. Intuition is something we all have, and again, is a part of the brain that can be exercised to be stronger. We've all had "hunches" about things, and when this happens, that is our intuition working.

Imagination is the ability to create and build pictures in the mind. We often think of artistic types of people as the only ones have much imagination, but that is not true. We all use imagination to varying degrees. Even something as simple as thinking about a new outfit you want to buy for a special event requires imagination. First, you picture how you want to look, and then you go out shopping looking for the pieces that will turn your picture into reality. When you hear the saying "in the mind's eye," that is referring to imagination. It is really the ability to "see" things that aren't really there yet.

Will is the ability to concentrate and focus. It is giving yourself a command and then following it. It is the power of control the mind has over its own actions. This is where "willpower" comes from. Will is telling yourself you are going to do (or not do) something, and then sticking with that decision regardless of what else happens. Often dieters are told they just need to have more willpower, however, we now know with weight that willpower alone is not nearly enough to effect lasting changes. (More about that as we go onto later chapters).

And finally, perception is really just your point of view. Your perception about anything is usually based in your previous experiences. For instance, I may perceive my boss as being a really unfair person because she didn't give me the raise I asked for; however a co-worker may perceive the exact same boss as being very fair because she did allow for a day off last month. Perception and opinion are often intertwined, and this can be where conflicts can arise, as one person's perception (or view) of a thing can be vastly different from another's. We can think of perception as the "lens through which we look at a subject" and each person's lens can be very different from another's. It is important to remember that we each have different perceptions, and you will become a master of getting along with people when you can start to look at the world through others' perceptions. You'll be surprised what you might see!

Now you have a better idea about the six lesser-known capabilities of the mind – memory, reason, will, imagination, perception, and intuition. And now that we have looked at the mind and what it is truly capable of, wouldn't you agree that is it far superior to even the most advanced computers available today? Perhaps sometime in the future, someone will invent a computer just as powerful (or maybe even more so) than our minds, but for today, the mind rules!

Now here's the paradox: when it's not fully engaged our mind can be our best ally, or our worst enemy.

And even though we have all this power available in our minds, the fact is that most of us spend a good deal of time on "auto pilot," going through our daily lives without being in the moment and without using our conscious minds. Instead relying on on habits, routine, and muscle memory. Given what we humans have accomplished without using our minds to their fullest potential at all times, just think what we could achieve if we did! The sky would be the limit!

Now here's the paradox: when it is not fully engaged our mind can be our best ally, or our worst enemy. The mind has power over each and every one of us, and thank goodness we have methods to determine whether this power is used for good or evil. And you are in luck, because The *Why Are You Weighting?* program is designed to help you get your mind working for you, as your greatest ally ever! Believe it or not, up to now, your mind most likely has not been working towards helping you at all, and in fact, may have been hindering you. Let's get a bit deeper into what I mean here.

What is the mind? Most of us have heard the idea that there are two parts to our minds, the conscious and the subconscious. However, do you really know the difference in terms of how the two different parts of the mind work? Let's examine this further because understanding how the two parts work, and using each part effectively, is so important with regard to ensuring that the *Why Are You Weighting?* program works.

Let's begin with looking at the conscious mind. The conscious mind is the part of your mind that you are aware of. It is where you do your "thinking." It is where you give yourself commands, such as "go to work," "take a vacation," and of course "reduce my weight". It is where you store data to be retrieved at a later time. It is where you figure out a math problem, or the best route to take on a road trip. It is where language comes from. It is the part of your mind that is working when you are reading or studying. It is the part of the mind that is being referred to when speaking of someone's intelligence. (Or lack of it.)

The conscious mind is truly what separates us from the beasts!

The conscious mind has the capacity to either accept or reject an idea, based on judgments you make. For instance, if someone were to say "the sky is green" your brain would hear these words, know they were not true, and then dismiss them. These words would have no real effect on you, because your conscious brain would reject them. At best, they would make you laugh, and wonder if the speaker had been drinking!

So, in this green-sky scenario, you realize that there is no truth to the idea, and no reason to accept and hold onto this misinformation. The conscious mind made a judgment, and decided this was rubbish, and not worth believing or storing. In a situation like this, when an idea is not accepted by the conscious, the brain doesn't store it — consciously or subconsciously. It is just "filtered out" and discarded.

The reverse of this is true, too. When an idea is accepted by the conscious mind, it is stored in the brain. In fact, this is how we learn. And the more often the conscious mind is presented with the same idea, and accepts it, the more often it gets stored and the more securely it is planted. You actually know this is true from your own experiences of learning. Most people are not very good at a new task (physical or mental) when they first start, but with constant repetition, it gets easier and the outcome gets better.

We store information on literally millions of things! How to add and subtract, how to read, how to eat, how to walk! Remember, these are all things that at one point in your life you didn't know how to do. The first few times you tried anything new, you probably failed, or at least performed badly. And yet, the more you did them (repetition), the easier they became. In fact most of these things now happen for you with very little thought. You just do them, and you do them well.

Now let's talk about the other part of the mind, the subconscious.

The subconscious mind is the part of your mind you are most likely unaware of. It too has many functions. For instance, it takes care of running our heart and lungs. Can you imagine how hard it would be if we had to actually think about keeping our hearts beating and our lungs inflating and deflating? I doubt we'd be able to get through a day and get anything done other than just staying alive!

Just as the subconscious keeps our hearts and lungs functioning every minute of every day, it is also running many of the rest of our activities, too. It can do this because the subconscious contains "programming" much the way a computer does. Just as a computer has an operating system which runs constantly in the background, we have an operating system running in the background of our minds! And our personal operating systems are found in our subconscious minds. We are all programmed for certain things. For instance, we are born programmed with the instructions that keep our heart and lungs functioning, along with most of our other bodily functions. And then later on, we add more programming on just about everything we do...how to walk, how to add and subtract, how to read, and even how to eat. There is an awful lot going on in the backgrounds of our minds in the area known as the subconscious.

And it is this background programming that really does run our lives. It controls not only on the things we don't have to think about, like breathing, but also many of the things we do need to think about. Our programming determines what types of foods we like, what types of people we like, even what type of clothes we like. It determines the type of person we'll end up with as a life partner and what we'll do for a living. Our programming also determines whether we are habitually punctual or late, organized or messy, fit or out of shape, rich or poor, and even slim or overweight.

So many things we think we control are really out of our conscious control.

It is estimated that about 95 percent of what we do each day is controlled by the subconscious and only 5 percent by the conscious. This means that 95 percent of our actions, our thoughts, our conversations, and even our outcomes, are being determined by the subconscious, all without us having any awareness that this is happening! Reread the previous two sentences; they are that important!

Our subconscious minds can really be thought of as our own personal "autopilot." And as you now know, for most of the time, the autopilot is really the one running the show.

So if 95 percent of everything we do is without our conscious awareness, you may ask how you can stop this. And I'm here to tell you that there is nothing you can do to stop this; it is the just the way we are designed to work. But don't despair.....

What you can do is work with the autopilot to effect changes. By knowing that the autopilot is the one leading the way, wouldn't you agree it makes sense that if we give the autopilot new or different information, we'll get different outcomes?

Now before we go on to learning how to effectively deal with our personal autopilots, let's look back at where our autopilots have already been. For instance, let's investigate where our autopilot originally got its programming. This is where things get really interesting!

In the first five years of our lives, our conscious brain is not fully developed, and so it has not yet mastered the ability to accept or reject a thought. Furthermore, because the conscious is not yet acting as an efficient "filter," most of what the mind is exposed to comes in, goes right past the not-yet-fully-functioning conscious, and gets stored in the subconscious. And our autopilots are there, soaking up everything that comes in.

Now think about what your life was like around you from birth to age five. Even though you won't remember much, if anything, from then, recall what you have heard from family members and friends who were around during that time. And if you have never thought about this, it would be worth the time to ask a few questions of those who would remember those years and what was happening then.

What were the people and situations like all around you from your birth to age 5? Were they happy times for those you were with, or unhappy? Were those people outspoken, or more of a quiet bunch? Were they open-minded and loved to learn, or more close-minded and rather opinionated? Did your parents treat each other nicely, or were they a meaner sort of couple? Did one or the other of your parents care for you daily or did they work leaving you with a friend, grandparent, babysitter or a child-care centre? Or maybe you were raised by one parent during this time. Did that parent say evil things about the other or were they friendly?

Were you plunked down in front of the TV all the time, or did someone spend time with you teaching you to read or playing games with you? Did you get yelled at if you made a mistake, or were your care-givers more forgiving sorts? Were you encouraged to be yourself, or were you pushed to be like someone else? Did you spend time in a city or in the country? Were you taken outside for activities, or did you spend most of your time indoors? Were creative pursuits encouraged, such as painting, dancing, or music? Or were you encouraged to spend your time on more academic things, like learning to read and write? Or were you left alone a lot of the time, with no direction at all?

I could on here for literally pages and pages, but I think you get the idea. There was A LOT going on around us every minute during the first five years of our lives, and we lacked the ability to decide what should have been store in our brains, and what didn't need to be. So we absorbed and stored just about everything.

If you spent much of your time alone as a young child, you may find as an adult that you simply must have a lot of alone time in order to feel like yourself, and as such, may choose a more solitary vocation such as accounting, where you don't have to interact with others to do your work. Conversely, if you spent a lot of your time in those first five years surrounded by other people, the adult version of you may only feel really comfortable when there are others around, and may then choose work where dealing with people is a big part of it, such as customer service or team-building.

If, as a child, you were encouraged to be creative and play, the adult version of you probably feels best when you are involved in creative pursuits, or otherwise having fun. This will determine what you like to do in your leisure hours. You would most likely end up taking painting, writing, or rug-hooking classes, and enjoy going to those classes because they are fun. Likewise, if you were encouraged to be more serious, as in "children should be seen and not heard," you may end up as an adult who is most comfortable in less "frivolous" pursuits and prefers reading as a leisure activity. These are just examples, and everyone is different, but I hope this gives you an idea of how our first five years of life really do have an effect on what we are going to be drawn towards as we mature.

> This borrowing of experience is better known as "listening to someone else's opinion."

This is why the first five years of a person's life are called the formative years. So much about who we ultimately turn out to be is determined in those few short years, because we were like a sponge, soaking up all that was going on around us. And remember, we had no way of filtering out all the good information from the bad, the true from the false, nor the bad situations and people from the good. We heard and saw all around us, and all of it had an impact on our minds.

Then, as we moved on past the age of five, the conscious became better and better at its filtering abilities. And a big part of how the conscious decides what to filter out, and what to let through, is based on experience. For instance, we reject the idea that the sky is green, because we know, from our previous experiences of looking at the sky, that it is blue.

And often, if we don't have an experience of our own to use a basis for this filtering, we will "borrow" someone else's experience to help us decide. This borrowing of experience is better known as "listening to someone else's opinion." We still do this even as adults. Think about the last time you were looking to make a major purchase, say a car or a home appliance. You most likely did some research beforehand. You may have searched the Internet and read what other people had to say about the product you were considering. You may have called a few friends and asked if they were happy with the brand they were using. And you took all this information in hand as you made your final decision. You would have felt a little more secure in your choice, since you could combine what you knew with others' experiences.

In other words, since you didn't have your own experiences to draw on, you listened to others' experiences and opinions, and acted based on those. In this particular example, it was a good thing to ask others before making your choice, because it helped you get the right model. (Or even just to avoid a bad model, if you got negative feedback about a certain brand.)

Now depending on the situation, listening to others can be either a positive or a negative thing to do. It really depends on the merits and credibility of the person giving you the opinion, and even what is going on in his or her life at the time. When listening to someone else's opinion, the more background info you have on the person, the better armed you are to know if the advice you are getting really has any merit.

There's an important point here we need to cover. Be aware that an opinion and a belief are interchangeable words. And most importantly, know that opinions and beliefs are not facts. For every belief or opinion someone holds, I guarantee that there is someone else whose opinion or belief is in exact opposition to the first person's opinion. Each may debate and discuss, trying to get the other to see and accept a particular view, sometimes even going into battle in an effort to get the other person to drop one belief and adopt a new one.

Opinions can be dangerous, because "someone else's opinion" is just what that person believes, and may not have any basis in fact whatsoever! Look at what people have believed over the years. Once, it was believed that the earth was flat. Once it was believed that women shouldn't vote. Once it was believed that slavery was okay. Once it was believed that humans would never fly, and certainly never get to the moon!

Today, every single one of these beliefs has been challenged! And like all beliefs, once they've been challenged, new beliefs begin to emerge. In today's world the Earth is round, women vote, slavery has been abolished, people fly everyday, and a few people have even been to the moon! What was believed 100 years ago is no longer believable! And while today we think of ourselves as enlightened and educated, much of what we believe to be true today will eventually turn out to be false. This has been true of every generation before us, and will be true for future generations as well.

Even ideas that are supported by science and thought of as fact can (and should) be challenged. While Sir Isaac Newton (the apple falling from the tree story) has often been called "the greatest scientist ever," and left us an impressive body of work known as Newtonian Mechanics, even some of his work has been challenged. In addition, there is now a field of study that would be completely foreign to Newton called Quantum Physics. This branch of physics looks at our world in new and different ways, and discoveries and theories in the field have turned out to have ramifications that go beyond pure science into the realms of philosophy and metaphysics.

It's important to keep in mind that there are facts that refer indisputably to what actually "is," such as the fact that the title of this book is Why Are You Weighting? and the fact that the chemical we call water is formed from the bond of two hydrogen atoms and one oxygen atom. However, many a fact is really just a belief that has yet to be successfully challenged. When a fact is successfully challenged, then it is no longer a fact, and will be replaced by the new fact, which again, will remain as fact until it is successfully challenged. But they are really just beliefs!

So what does all this have to do with releasing weight and keeping it off? Ah, the million dollar question: *Why Are You Weighting?*

We've all had experiences or people in our lives that have lead us to believe certain things about ourselves and our bodies. Everyone has had this, although sometimes it is easier to understand this by looking at others. Think of the people you know...is there one who seems to you to have a distorted self-image? For instance, you may have a friend who you think is really smart, but he'll deny it, and say he is not very intelligent at all. This may stem from him having had a teacher or parent who told him he was stupid, or that he wouldn't amount to anything. You know it is not true, yet he firmly believes it.

You may know someone you think has a terrific figure, yet when you compliment her, she'll immediately point out her flaws. You look at her and see a knockout, yet when she looks in the mirror she sees a very different picture. Again, this could be because someone told her that she had a bad figure, so when she looks at herself, that is what she sees. You know that she looks great; however, you can't get her to see herself that way. She believes something different about herself than you do.

The same is true in reverse. Just as we see others differently than they see themselves, it is important to realize that often, others see us differently than we see ourselves. In other words, often people have different beliefs about us than we have about ourselves.

And they are just beliefs, which means that they can be challenged, and often disproved.

For instance, you may believe that you are clumsy. You may believe that you are sick often. You may believe that you can't release weight. You may believe that you hate your body, because your thighs/tummy/arms/back are too fat. You may believe that you cannot do certain things, like exercise, or dance, or ice skate or.....

Some of the beliefs may have come from your experiences. Say you've tried a few times to ice skate, and just can't seem to get the hang of it. You may form the belief "I can't ice skate." Or, some of your beliefs about yourself may actually have come from someone else's belief about you. For instance, when you were learning to ride a bike, a friend may have said, "Oh you are clumsy!" just as you fell and embarrassed yourself, so you start to believe you are a clumsy person, even though really, you just had a clumsy moment.

If you really wanted to ice skate, you could still learn, even today. With the right teacher and a commitment to getting the hang of it (i.e., practice), it wouldn't be long before you were gliding around the rink like a pro! Your belief of "I can't ice skate" would be replaced with "I can ice-skate" — in other words, a new belief!

I've said it before and I'm going to repeat it here. Beliefs are not necessarily grounded in fact!

So now, how to apply this knowledge to our bodies?

Let's look at some of the beliefs you may currently hold about your body, at least with relation to your weight. Here are a few common ones I've heard people say over and over again.

Everything I eat turns to fat.
My family is fat, so I am too.
I can't exercise because I'm too fat.
My butt has always been too big.
I'll always be fat because I like to eat.

Often we don't really realize we are even referring to our bodies when we make statements like this. So really what is being said here is:

I believe that everything I eat turns to fat on my body.
My family members all have fat bodies, so I believe that
I have to have one, too.
I believe that my fat body can't move.
I believe that my body will always have a big butt.
I believe that my body will always be fat because I like to eat.

Using the examples above, what beliefs do you hold about your own body? Take a few minutes and think about this. I think you'll be surprised what you come up with. Your answers may be like the examples above, or they may be very different. But I know that somewhere inside of you, you hold some type of beliefs about your body. We all do.

And if you have any of these types of thoughts repeatedly, these thoughts are going to get stored in your brain. Each time you think, "I'm fat," your brain takes that message, and re-enforces it. Think it often enough and it becomes part of your subconscious. And since we know that the autopilot lives in the subconscious, and that our autopilot is really our programming, you can begin to see how you are actually programming yourself to be fat!

This is because your autopilot, now programmed with "I'm fat," will actually look for ways to keep you fat! And remember, all this is happening without your conscious awareness of it.

So even though you go on a diet and vow this time to really stick with it, because you're actually programmed on a subconscious level to be fat, you will end up sabotaging yourself each and every time. And you know this has happened when you find yourself thinking, "Why did I _____?" Just fill in the blank with whatever it was you vowed you wouldn't do, such as eat the cake, have a second helping, skip your workout, choose the cream sauce, etc., etc., etc! The answer is always, always, because you are programmed to be/stay fat.

In order to effect any permanent changes in our weight, we must deal with our beliefs about our bodies, in order to positively change our autopilots and our programming. If you don't attend to this, anything else you do will be short-lived at best. You will end up falling back into old habits, and getting the same old results.

So now it is time to form some new, positive beliefs about your body. Now we are going to work on reprogramming how you think about your body. We are going to reprogram the brain (your autopilot) to think of your body as slim and healthy. And doesn't it make sense to you that the autopilot of a slim, healthy body will have a different guidance system than the autopilot of an overweight, unhealthy body?

One of the major reasons most people gain back the weight they've lost is that they never updated their brain and autopilot to match their new body! And since the autopilot runs us, if it isn't brought up-to-date, it will continue to run the body as it was, not as it is.

So, starting right now, right this minute, you are going to begin thinking of yourself as slim and healthy, regardless of what you currently weigh. It doesn't matter whether you are 2 pounds or 200 pounds from your ideal weight, you are going to change the way you think about yourself, and when you do this repeatedly, you will change your autopilot.

And to do this, we are going to use a proven technique called *affirmations.* An affirmation is a positive statement you repeat over and over and over again to yourself until you actually start to believe it because it gets programmed into your subconscious and into your autopilot. An affirmation is always written in the present tense, even though sometimes this can seem like quite a stretch of the truth! That is because the subconscious is always dealing in the right now — not the future, not the past, but right now. So it is important that your affirmations are in the present tense. If you make them future-dated, such as "I will" or "I am going to," you will not get the results you are looking for.

And a good affirmation will start with the words "I am so happy and grateful now that" because you want to set up a feeling of happiness with what you are working towards, and it keeps you in the present tense.

Now, you may want to be slim to feel better, or perhaps to look better, or maybe you want this so that your favourite activities become easier. Whatever your reason is, you are going to incorporate this into your affirmation. So your affirmation may sound like this: "I am so happy and grateful now that I am at my ideal body weight and in perfect health...I feel great!" Or, it may sound more like this: "I am so happy and grateful now that I am at my ideal body weight, and I look awesome! I wear attractive, tailored clothing that looks great on me!" It could also sound something like this: "I am so happy and grateful now that I am at my ideal body weight, and I have the energy of a child! I am able to dance and swim with ease, I am so graceful!"

I know for many people, saying these affirmations, especially when in the present tense, can feel ridiculous. You may feel like you are lying to yourself, because your statement seems so far away from the current reality. However, you are just going to have to trust me on this one. Keep saying (and thinking) your affirmations many, many times a day, and you will begin to see "miracles" happen. If you feel really silly or foolish, do these when you are alone. It can really help speed up the process if you can say your affirmation aloud, facing yourself in the mirror. This will help bridge the gap between what you are thinking about yourself and what you are seeing of yourself.

And as you are repeating your affirmation, it is important that you begin to feel what it is like to live in your slim body. At first, you will have to consciously work on creating these "slim" feelings, but again, the more you do this, the more you are going to feel this way without any conscious effort. And that is when the exponential leaps in progress happen.

HERE ARE A COUPLE OF EXAMPLES:

IF YOU ARE AFFIRMING how much better your slim body feels, then imagine yourself in situations where you are reminded of this. Imagine getting onto a plane or in a car and doing up the seatbelt with ease. Imagine going for a long walk with your back being pain-free. Imagine being able to breathe easily and move about without getting winded. Imagine the waistband of your pants being comfortable. Really feel how good your slim body feels.

IF YOU ARE AFFIRMING what you look like, use your imagination to see and feel yourself wearing a new outfit. Really get into this! Imagine all the details of your outfit, right down to what accessories you would have. In your mind's eye, see yourself wearing your outfit, in a suitable situation. See yourself moving around in your new clothes. See people complimenting your taste and style. Really feel how awesome it feels to be looking this good!

AND IF YOU ARE AFFIRMING your ability to do activities, then imagine yourself actually doing these activities. If dancing is your thing, then picture your slim self dancing and twirling around! Being lifted effortlessly by your partner, and then gracefully going into a dip! Perhaps skiing is your passion. If so, imagine yourself swooshing down the slopes effortlessly, easily flying over moguls and creating great sprays of snow! Maybe you just want to be able to keep up with your children or grandchildren....so imagine yourself playing with them, with lots of energy to spare. Imagine being able to easily pick them up, or running around the baseball field. Really feel what it is like to move so effortlessly.

AND REGARDLESS OF WHAT you are picturing, put a smile on your face as you do this. In fact, on both your faces...your real one, and the one in your imagination. This will help to move your body into a "feel-good" state. And the better you are feeling, the quicker your brain will accept the reprogramming, resulting in your autopilot thinking and acting like a slim person's autopilot.

So I want you stop right now and just try this. Sit quietly and close your eyes. Begin to see yourself in your slim body, doing or wearing or being what you want. Really focus on how good this feels...how good it feels to wear the outfit, or to be healthy, or to be energetic. And remember, smile on both the inside and the outside!

And don't be concerned if it feels like you are lying to yourself! This is normal. This feeling will go away as you continue to do the affirmations. Just trust the process. And whenever thoughts like "this isn't true" or "you liar" pop into your head, just re-focus on your imagination and your affirmation. The more you do this, the easier it becomes, and you'll have fewer and fewer distracting thoughts.

I cannot stress how powerful this process is!

So, for the next 30 days, you are going to take a minimum of 10 minutes, morning and evening, and do your affirmations. You are going to affirm your slim, healthy body! And as you do your affirmations, you are going to vividly imagine yourself in various situations in your slim, healthy body. Really, really visualize in your mind. Have fun with this! Be outrageous! It's your day dream, so do what you really want with it because the sky's the limit!

Really commit to doing this, and don't let anything get in your way!

I guarantee you that the way you think about your body will really start to change, and that is how your body will change, by changing the way you think. It really is that simple, and there truly is no other way to effect permanent changes.

Chapter 4 Summary

- Your mind can be your best friend or your worst enemy.
- What you currently believe to be true may not be true. A belief is not a fact.
- Affirmations work to reprogram our subconscious, and must always be in present tense.
- Smile and really feel good as you work through this.

Check out www.WhyAreYouWeighting.com
for more ideas on affirmations.

_____

_____

_____

_____

_____

CHAPTER 5
Paradigms

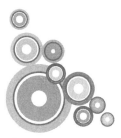

Chapter 5 – Paradigms

SO WHAT IS A Paradigm? (Pronounced "pear-ah-dime") And what does it have to do with weight? A lot, is the short answer, and the long answer is found in the rest of this chapter!

First, let's look at what a paradigm is. I looked up at least 10 different definitions, and the one that I think offers the easiest explanation is that a "paradigm is a multitude of habits." We all have paradigms in every aspect of our lives. We have family paradigms, work paradigms, health paradigms, political paradigms, relationship paradigms, personal paradigms....the list is almost endless!

A paradigm can also be looked at as the (often unwritten) set of rules and regulations belonging to an individual, a family, a company, a government, or a culture. When you think about it, what is a rule really, other than a directive about habits — habits that will and will not be tolerated?

Let's look at a couple of these paradigms from the "habit" side and let's start with the family paradigm, since all of us have had some experience dealing with families! All families have habits. It may be your familial habit that Dad sits at the head of the table, Mom to his right, and the kids in the other seats. Dad would never think of sitting anywhere but at the head, that's just the way it is, it's that family's habit or paradigm. In fact, often habits turn into rules. After a while, Dad begins to think of his sitting at the head of the table to be the family rule, and no one dares challenge it!

There will also be paradigms regarding the inter-relationships of the various family members. For example, big brother always teases little brother, and then little brother turns around and torments even-littler sister. Little sister then runs to play with her dolls in order to escape. Mom yells at big brother, who then leaves the house, slamming the door on his way out. A scenario like this is rarely a one-time event, but rather is usually repeated many times in a month, and in fact, becomes a habit played out amongst the various family members. Basically the paradigm goes like this...Mom always ends up yelling, big brother always ends up leaving, little brother always ends up tormenting his sister, and little sister always ends up playing with her dolls. These actions have become habits.

Think of all the habits or paradigms that exist around an office. The boss may think that it is necessary to have a Monday morning meeting, so that becomes the habit. The boss may also declare that it is necessary that everyone be dressed in formal work attire, rather than a more business-casual look, so dressing up becomes the habit. The workers may decide to celebrate everyone's birthdays in the office, so having a cake and singing Happy Birthday becomes the habit.

So the office paradigm becomes "we always have a Monday morning meeting, everyone dresses in formal business wear, and we always celebrate everyone's birthdays." Again, all these actions have become habits, and some of them even become rules. "You must wear formal attire" becomes the rule for this office, even though there are other offices and other companies that allow more casual dressing, without any detriment to their businesses.

A few paragraphs back, I mentioned culture and that there are paradigms in each culture. In fact, any culture (corporate, ethnic, religious, etc.) really is just a way of doing things according to a certain set of rules, or in a certain way (habit). And while we all come from different backgrounds and cultures, if you think about your culture, you will realize that you most definitely have rules about how to behave and how to do things and even how to think! Some cultures are more rigid, and some more relaxed; however, each and every culture has some set of rules. That's one of the reasons we all feel more comfortable in our own cultures, because we know the rules and what's expected of us, and are therefore less likely to do anything to embarrass ourselves or others!

Some cultures favour capitalism; some favour a more socialistic approach. Some cultures believe in equality amongst the sexes, and some believe one sex is superior over the other. Some cultures value aging and wisdom, and some cultures believe that the elderly have nothing of value to offer. Some cultures idolize the very thin, and some cultures adore the more rotund members. Some cultures promote meat-eating, while others are vegetarian-based. This list could go on for pages!

Often a paradigm within any group of people will say that if you don't do something a certain way, you are doing it incorrectly. Yet other groups of people follow completely different sets of rules, and they still get by. I point this out to you to help you begin to understand that a paradigm, while often preached as the law, is really not. For everyone who holds a certain paradigm, there will be another person who holds the complete opposite paradigm.

So now that you know what a paradigm is, let's look at how they work, and what they have to do with weight and health.

Paradigms are stored in our subconscious brain and are the rules that our own personal autopilots follow. In the previous chapter we looked at how ideas and concepts get planted in the subconscious, both during and after the first five formative years of life. We also learned about how our subconscious (aka our autopilot) directs 95 percent of what is going on in our lives, so you begin to understand why it is so important to really examine the paradigms that are running your life. The good news is that you can change them if they are not really helping you get to where you want to be.

Now I need to stress something here. Changing a paradigm is not an easy feat. It is not impossible by any means, but also it is not easy. However, in any area of your life, literally any area (personal, professional, health, wealth, etc.), if you are not getting the results you want, you must examine your paradigms and then change them, in order to change your outcome. This you can take to the bank!

And so I would like us to examine the differences in paradigms between the healthy, slim population, and the overweight population. By highlighting the differences between these two groups, you will start to see how your paradigms (habits) are playing into your results, both good and bad! The following are just some simple examples. You may recognize your own thinking in some of these, and/or you may discover you have others not listed here.

Overweight paradigm: It doesn't matter what I eat, I'll gain weight anyway.
Healthy, slim paradigm: I choose foods that are healthy, knowing that what I eat does matter.

Overweight paradigm: Exercise is hard, I hate it, and I don't want to do it.
Healthy, slim paradigm: Exercise is good for my body, and makes me feel good. I love to exercise.

Overweight paradigm: It's ok to eat (large amounts of food) late at night.
Healthy, slim paradigm: I avoid eating after 8 p.m., and if I am really hungry, I'll just eat a light snack.

Overweight paradigm: A second helping is the norm.
Healthy, slim paradigm: A single serving is the norm.

Overweight paradigm: Deep-fried foods are really tasty, and not really that bad for me.
Healthy, slim paradigm: Deep-fried foods are not that tasty, and they can be harmful to my health.

Overweight paradigm: I have a creamy dessert with every meal.
Healthy, slim paradigm: I only have rich desserts on special occasions. Normally, I just have fruit as dessert.

Overweight paradigm: I eat everything on my plate.
Healthy, slim paradigm: I eat to the point of satisfaction, and then just stop.

Overweight paradigm: I'll make myself feel better by eating.
Healthy, slim paradigm: I'll make myself feel better by calling a friend.

Overweight paradigm: I'm bored; I think I'll get something to eat.
Healthy, slim paradigm: I'm bored; I think I'll go to a for a walk.

Overweight paradigm: When I am preparing food, I'll just have a couple of tastes as I go!
Healthy, slim paradigm: I don't sample or taste when I am preparing food.

Get the idea? Overweight people just think differently than healthy, slim people.

And you can see how each one of these examples, based on the thinking, that the actions the overweight person is going to take are going to be radically different than the actions of the slim person.

So you begin to see how what you think about leads to what actions you will take. And it is not a big jump to realize that the actions you take are going to lead to the results you get. Let's examine further how our thinking (a.k.a. our paradigms) determines our results or outcomes.

Before we go on, I must point out that the subject of paradigms is so important, I cannot stress it enough. Joel Barker, the author of some famous business books, is quoted as saying, "To ignore the power of paradigms to influence your judgment is to put yourself at risk when exploring the future."

Although I am sure Barker was referring to business when he uttered those words, let's paraphrase this quote with the idea of our weight in mind. "To ignore how your thoughts about weight and weight reduction are affecting you (e.g., your judgments about what to eat, how and when to exercise, etc.) is to put yourself at risk of not achieving what you want (your ideal body weight) in the future."

So how do we go about changing our paradigms? There are only two ways! The first is through an emotional impact. To look at this from a weight perspective, this type of change (paradigm shift) might come if you were told by your doctor that your weight has lead to heart disease. This news would fill you with the emotion of fear, and fear is a strong motivator for change! So, this type of news might cause you to make the permanent changes in food choices and lifestyle that could restore your health. In other words, you would form new food and lifestyle paradigms because you were emotionally affected by the bad health news.

Now I am not suggesting you need to wait until you get some really bad news to make the necessary changes! The "emotional impact" method of paradigm change is the rarer (and more uncontrollable) of the two forms, so let's look at the more common method.

Reprogramming our subconscious minds is the only way to effect permanent and lasting change. The only way!

The other way to shift your paradigms, (your ideas) is through the constant repetition of a new idea in order to replace the old idea. Remember, paradigms are stored in our subconscious, and they run the show! So wouldn't you agree it makes sense that by re-programming our subconscious minds (our autopilots) we can head in a different direction? In fact, as I have previously mentioned, it is the only way to effect permanent and lasting changes. The only way!

This is really what is behind the affirmations that we started in the previous chapter. An affirmation, repeated often, is the "constant repetition" that we need to maintain our ideal weight. In the last chapter we looked at affirmations for changing the way we feel about and see ourselves. Now we are going to look at changing our paradigms for food and exercise.

Here are some affirmations to use before you begin to eat, whether it is a meal or a snack. Pick a couple that sound good to you, and begin to use them immediately, even (and especially) if they are not exactly "true" at this point!

I AM SO HAPPY AND GRATEFUL NOW THAT I...

- am eating smaller portions of food
- am only having one plate of food
- am making healthy food choices
- am eating to fuel my body, not to deal with emotions
- am eating like a slim person
- am honouring my body by giving it what it needs and no more

BECAUSE I FEEL SO GOOD WHEN I DO!

These affirmations, when repeated often enough, are going to move past your conscious, and get stored in your subconscious, where they will become part of your autopilot. And once your autopilot has adopted them, they will become part of your programming. This means that they will become the rules that the autopilot uses when it is directing that 95 percent of what you do everyday!

And here are some affirmations to use when you are about to start moving your body (i.e., exercise). And if you can't wrap your head around actually exercising at this stage, it is even more important to say these affirmations, as they will move your thinking into a more positive view about exercise, which will cause your autopilot to get you moving one way or the other!

I AM SO HAPPY AND GRATEFUL NOW THAT I...

- am able to move effortlessly and gracefully
- am able to give my body what it needs through regular exercise
- am creating my ideal body
- love exercising
- am able to move my body
- have added movement to my routine

BECAUSE I FEEL SO GOOD WHEN I DO!

You want to get an appreciation or even love of exercise programmed into your autopilot to create a new exercise paradigm. If your autopilot hates exercising, it is going to be really difficult for you to develop an exercise habit that sticks. You may do ok for a couple of weeks, but you will begin to falter, and eventually you will fall off the exercise bandwagon altogether. You must program your autopilot into liking exercise, and once that happens, you will find that you actually begin to like exercise, and will get some just about every day, whether you think about it consciously or not.

Practice these over and over and over again. And then practice them some more! You are working against years and decades of the old programming, so this is going to take time. Don't expect overnight results however, do expect results. You are not going to undo 20, 30, even 40 or more years of old thinking in just a day, or even a week. It is going to take some time. But time is going to pass regardless, so isn't it exciting to know that you can change your future and your outcomes? That the next five years don't have to be like the last five years? (Or even fifty years for that matter!)

There are ways to increase the effectiveness of your affirmations. One important way is to really put some positive emotion into them. Remember in the previous chapter I talked about smiling both on the inside and the outside when you are saying an affirmation? Practicing your affirmations must not feel like drudgery, or like just another item on your to-do list. Because if it does, I guarantee you these affirmations will not work. You must feel good about doing them and good while you are doing them!

However, by saying them with a smile on your face, and with enthusiasm and excitement in your voice, these affirmations will work, I guarantee you! And remember, no matter how big the distance between where you are now and where you want to be, no matter how much you initially feel like a liar or a fake when saying these things, say them anyway! Affirmations are your secret weapon on the road to your ideal weight. They change your paradigms, which changes your autopilot, which changes your actions, which changes your results.

In addition to paradigms around food, exercise, and our bodies, there are a couple of other areas we should look at with regard to our paradigms. And believe it or not, one of the things you will need to examine is the thoughts you hold about those who are already slim, regardless of whether this is their natural state or they have just reduced their weight. In my journey, I came to realize that on some level, I resented "thin people," especially those who were wearing the type of clothes I longed to be able to wear. I was filled with jealousy when I was faced with someone slim and stylish! I love clothes and always have, and thought it was so unfair that healthy-weight people should be able to look so good, when I didn't. I used to scrutinize their slim bodies, looking for something that I could criticize (in my mind) in order to make myself feel better. Does any of this sound familiar to you? Don't gloss over this. Really examine your thoughts on this, because it is that important.

The negative thoughts in you might be stirred up about something other than how they look. You may discover that you are jealous about the fact that someone can do an activity that you feel you can't do because of your weight. You may discover that you have the green-eyed monster show up when you see a slim person in a happy relationship, believing that a good relationship can't happen for you because of your weight. Or maybe you told yourself that only slim people get promotions and all the good jobs. Pay attention whenever you find yourself feeling those negative emotions, (jealousy, envy, even anger) and commit to uncovering the reasons why.

This is important, because if you are holding on to any type of negative emotional thinking about others who are slim, while at the same time hoping and wishing for a slim body yourself, you are creating a mixed message in your mind. Your autopilot won't know which way to steer you, because you haven't been clear about what you want. On one hand, your autopilot gets the message that "slim makes you feel bad" (i.e., jealousy about others) and then on the other hand gets the message that "slim is what I want." The result of this is massive confusion in your mind! And your autopilot, thinking that slim equals bad is going to do everything in its power to do good, translating this into overweight equals good.

Do you see how this works? So what do we do about it?

Again, it comes down to changing your thinking, your paradigm. From this moment forth, every time you are faced with someone slim and stylish/active/happy, etc., who brings out these negative thoughts and feelings in you, STOP and replace those thoughts with something more in line with what you really want. And don't judge yourself for thinking the "bad" thought; that is just wasted energy! Simply notice that you had the thought, and then immediately replace it.

I have learned to silently bless or praise the person who has what I want, and this sets up a very different reaction for my autopilot to follow. By thinking a thought like "Wow, I love what that slim looking woman is wearing; she looks terrific!" I set up the idea that slim equals terrific, and that, coupled with my desire to be slim myself, is a single, straight forward message, without any mix-ups. The idea that slim equals good is reinforced in my subconscious, and my autopilot gets to work on creating that for me!

THIS IS A SIMPLE, YET POWERFUL CONCEPT!

Here are some examples of more positive thinking that you can use to replace any negative thoughts:

• I love how that slim person looks so fit and agile!

- I love how that slim person looks so stylish and looks so good!

- I love that that slim person is in a great relationship!

And be sure to put some excitement and enthusiasm into your thoughts! If you are able, it is always great to actually tell the person your great, positive thoughts. Everyone loves to receive praise, and it is never, ever a bad thing to offer someone a sincere compliment.

You may have noticed that there are certain people or situations that cause you to really want to eat too much or to skip your workout. These types of reactions are again an example of your paradigms. You may believe that because someone or something annoyed you, that gives you permission to overeat or not exercise. This is just a habit, and when you change the habit, the results change.

Or maybe you always overeat when you are with a certain group of friends, food being your only common element. Or perhaps you get so stressed at work that you routinely decide to skip your end-of-day workout when you have had a bad day. In either of these situations, or any others you may run across that are similar, it is again your paradigms that cause the "often repeated behaviour."

It is important to pay attention to the people and situations that trigger you to move in the wrong direction. What's the wrong direction? Any direction that takes you further away from what you want. If you are wanting to release some weight, and then you go and overeat, or skip your exercise, that is moving in the wrong direction. And I guarantee you it is your paradigms causing this to happen. You simply must notice what causes you to move in the wrong direction, and then change your thoughts!

Success, or a lack of it, all begins, and ends, with your thoughts!

And the last, but certainly not the least, thoughts we are going to cover here are the thoughts you hold about your own body. There are two areas we need to pay attention to, if we are to easily maintain a healthy weight for the rest of our lives.

The first is how you think about your body. Notice the thoughts that go through your mind each day with regard to your physical self. Are you loving and compassionate towards your body, or judgmental and critical? Monitor your self-talk and see which way you speak to yourself about your body. When you look in the mirror, what do you see and what do you think about what you see? For instance, do you focus on the areas that you really like, that you are confident about, and have thoughts like, "I have lovely shoulders" or "I really like my legs"? Or do you immediately go the "problem areas," and focus on what you are less confident of? Do you find yourself thinking along the lines of "my thighs are so jiggley" or "boy, I look awful"?

What message are you sending yourself? One of love and acceptance, or one of judgment and criticism?

No one, not even the super models or super-athletes, has a "perfect" body.

So here's more to add to your homework, every single day. Every time you look into a mirror, pay attention to the thoughts that appear. If these thoughts are anything even slightly critical, replace them by focusing on some part of your physical self that you do like. And then give yourself a sincere compliment. You may like your eyes, or your hair, or your hands, or your feet, or your ankles! Surely there is something about yourself that you do like. Focus on that, and then think "Wow, I have beautiful _____! Just look at _____, it's gorgeous!"

And if you really, truly don't have an area of your physical body that you can honestly say you like, then this just proves that you are being critical and judgmental with yourself. And it's time to stop!

So regardless of whether you just discovered that you are very judgmental about yourself or just mildly so, it's time to plant some seeds of positivity, and then nurture those seeds until they grow into complete and full self-acceptance.

One of the strongest reasons I think we usually gain back the released weight is that we (our conscious and our autopilots) don't really think of ourselves as "ideal weight" people, regardless of what the scale may be saying. We don't take the time to update our autopilots about the new version of ourselves, and so we continue to think the thoughts that the older version of us used to think.

I had a big epiphany about this a few years ago while sitting at a beach in Mexico. I was sitting there, literally weighing the least I had ever weighed as an adult (in fact less than most of my years as a teen, too!) and I found myself trying to cover up my body, thinking that everyone on the beach would be looking at me and judging me for being so fat. I also found myself looking at the overweight people on the beach, seeing what types of bathing suits and cover-ups they were wearing, to get ideas for myself! But I wasn't even fat then, I was normal-weighted! So what was really happening?

I know now that what was going on for me that day (and many other days like it) was that I hadn't reprogrammed my autopilot to truly think of myself and see myself at my new weight. In my mind, I was still using the old "fat pictures" when thinking of myself. I was still programmed to think and act as I had when I was a large woman, and for me that meant trying to cover up at the beach so that no one would see my fat and make fun of me or judge me for it.

Why does this happen for us? It all has to do with our paradigms. I can't say it often enough! Everything has to do with our paradigms! In my case, my paradigms hadn't changed to match the new me. And I realized that if I didn't change them, they sure weren't going to change themselves. After all, I had been at this new weight for over a year, and yet my autopilot was still operating on old info.

I am so grateful for this day at the beach, because it got me thinking about how to change my thinking! This turned out to be one of the pivotal moments in my life-long journey with my weight. And if I hadn't have had this epiphany, I know now that I would have never have been able to maintain my new weight. Like every other time before, I would have ended up watching the scales getting higher and higher, while my self-esteem plummeted lower and lower.

So it's important that we change our programming about what we look like and how we see ourselves. And as with the other paradigms we have worked on in this program, it is constant repetition that will do the trick.

So let me ask you, "How badly do you want to get a handle on your weight?"

At this point, you may feel like rolling your eyes and thinking "More affirmations? More homework? This is too much!" So let me ask you, "How badly do you want to get a handle on your weight? How badly do you want to be in an ideal weight body forever?" Nothing worth having in life comes easily. Do you actually think it is easier to deprive yourself of food for months on end (dieting) than it is to spend 10 to 20 minutes a day looking at yourself in a mirror and repeating certain phrases over and over again? Watch your answers here; they will reveal a lot about your paradigms!

To begin changing your programming about what you look like and how you see yourself, you are going to need a picture of yourself at your ideal weight. If that is you now, great, get someone to snap a fantastic picture of you right away! If you are currently heavier than you'd like to be, find a fairly recent (within the last couple of years) photo of yourself where you are at a more desirable weight. And if there isn't one, don't worry; you are going to make one!

Find a picture of someone with a body type similar to yours who is at the ideal weight. Be sure this is realistic. If you are broad-shouldered and have short legs, look for someone who fits that description, not a thin, leggy model type. If you've never been ideal-weighted as an adult, then really think about what your body type would look like at its ideal weight, and hunt through various magazines to find it. Be sure to look beyond the fashion and glamour magazines so that you get a good cross-section of real bodies at real weights. After all, striving to have a body like an underweight model is not a healthy ideal either. And remember, most (all?) of the pictures in the fashion and glamour magazines have had tons and tons of airbrushing and touch ups done to them to make the models look perfect! No one in real life looks like the models in the magazines, not even the models themselves! Don't set yourself up for failure by choosing an unrealistic, impossible ideal.

Okay, so now you have your ideal body weight picture. If you are using someone else's body for this, or if the picture is of you but was taken so long ago that your face in the picture doesn't really look like you at all now, then I want you to cut off the face in the picture, then replace the face in the picture with a more recent, nice shot of your face. You are going to be looking at this picture every day for quite a while, and I want your brain to instantly recognize the face as yours, so that the connection is made that the body is yours too!

Get five or more copies made of this picture. You are going to take this picture and put it in places where you will see it many times a day. For instance, tape one to your computer monitor, put one up in the bathroom, hang another in the kitchen, tape one to your closet door, and get one laminated and carry it around in your pocket. Be sure to place them where you will just naturally run into them during your usual routines. It's important that you repeatedly spend some time every 24 hours looking at it. And as we have learned, it is of utmost importance to feel good, really good, as you gaze upon this version of yourself. You want to bring up the great feelings that being at this ideal weight have caused in the past or will cause very soon. Think about how proud you are of your success, how easily it has all happened, how great it feels to wear really well-fitting clothes.

Do not allow yourself to slide down into negative thinking. If thoughts like "I'll never look like this!" or "Who am I kidding?" or "Why did I let myself go?" pop up, just notice them, and then replace them with positive thoughts. If you are so far down the spiral of negativity that being positive is too big a stretch, just think. "This is a current picture of me." At least this thought is neutral. And then work towards being able to think more positive thoughts.

Now it's time to turn these positive thoughts into affirmations! Say them out loud every time you look at this picture of yourself. (You can also think them to yourself if the situation is one where you can't say them out loud.) Here are a couple of ideas for affirmations. Use these or make up your own. "I am so happy, grateful, and proud now that I am easily living at my ideal weight!" or "I am so happy and grateful now that I am at my ideal weight, and I can do physical activities with ease and grace!" or "I am so happy and grateful now that I am at my ideal weight and my clothes look and feel great!"

Really pay attention to your autopilot during this, and if anything along the lines of "You don't really look like this, who are you kidding?" comes up, just notice the thought, and release it. Don't dwell on it, or give it anymore energy. Stay focused on the outcome — on what you look and feel like at your ideal weight. We really are working on brainwashing your autopilot into permanently seeing you as an ideal-weight person. When you are an ideal-weight person you are a person who is happy and you feel so good about yourself and your body that your autopilot ends up working everyday to maintain this state for you. And when you have achieved this level, you will say "Wow, maintaining my weight is so easy! I just never think about it any more!" and this will be your new reality!

One last note on "brainwashing." We have all been brainwashed to some degree or another; it's part of the human process of learning and growing up. So the tip for success is to re-brainwash yourself, using ideas that will actually get you to where you want to be. Again, it is the constant repetition of an idea, impressed on the subconscious, over and over and over again that will brainwash you into success!

Start doing your affirmations today! Start loving yourself today! Start loving others who have what you want today! Start having a strong mental picture of yourself at your ideal weight. And just watch what starts to happen for you...you will be amazed!

Chapter 5 Summary

- Paradigms are sets of unwritten rules that govern our lives.
- Constant repetition is required to shift a paradigm.
- Overweight people think differently than ideal weight people.
- Notice all your positive attributes and talents and start loving yourself.

Be sure to join our site at www.WhyAreYouWeighting.com and interact with the other members as we all work to shift our paradigms!

_____

_____

_____

_____

_____

"Affirmations are like prescriptions for certain aspects of yourself you want to change."

Jerry Frankhauser
From a "Chicken to an Eagle."

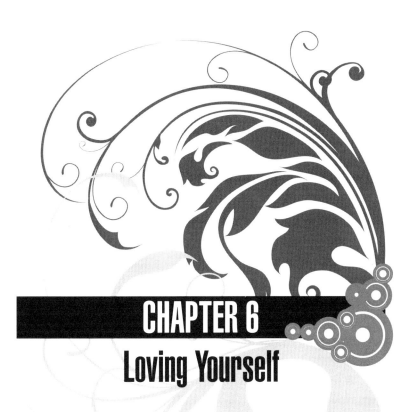

CHAPTER 6
Loving Yourself

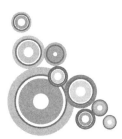

Chapter 6 — Loving Yourself

I BET THERE ARE all kinds of things you love. People, food, places, ideas, music, sleeping, pets, books, movies, nature, architecture, poetry, sports....the list is endless. And while none of us loves all things, we all have things we love.

Now here's a question for you. Do you love yourself?

What was your first thought when you read the question about loving yourself?

Was it something about loving yourself being wrong? Wrong, because to love yourself would be conceited? Wrong, because what would others think? Wrong, because you don't think of yourself as a lovable person? Wrong, because no one else loves you? Wrong, because people shouldn't just walk around loving themselves? Wrong, because..?

No matter what reason there is that you may believe that self-love is wrong, that reason is wrong!

You are a magnificent being! You are worthy of being loved, no matter what anyone else may have ever told you. And the first step to being loved is to really love and accept yourself. Fully embrace yourself, all of yourself.

Now, this may not be easy for you to hear. Your life story may involve people and situations that tried to tell you that weren't loved, that you didn't matter, or that you weren't worth it. Most likely, these were ideas you picked up during your formative years, in the first five years of your life. Unfortunately, some of the people around you may have deliberately tried to "bring you down" because they felt down themselves. Or you may have just picked up on some negative energy going on in your world, and interpreted it as being about you, leaving you feeling negative about yourself.

I am here to tell you none of this is true, not one word. No matter how far from ideal-weighted you are, no matter what you may have thought or said about yourself, and certainly no matter what others have said to you, or done to you, none of this is true. You may not believe me at this point, but we are going to challenge your beliefs. And as we have learned, a challenged belief leads to new beliefs. Then you are going to build new beliefs about yourself — beliefs which are empowering and uplifting, and that will help you move more quickly and easily toward your desires!

Back in Chapter 4 we talked about how our subconscious gets programmed. And one of the most important things that gets programmed into our subconscious is how we think about ourselves — our self-esteem.

Now, let's go back to our first five years of life. Chances are you had siblings or other children around you. How do children talk to each other? Usually not in the nicest manner! "You're stupid" or "You're ugly" are common childhood phrases that get thrown around in the playground regularly. And when you were with your parents, doing what children do, on a number of occasions you may have been told "You're a bad girl/boy." As you heard these phrases repeatedly over the years, these messages got stored in the subconscious, because your young brain did not have the capacity to decide if there was truth to these statements. Over time, the ideas that you are stupid, or ugly, or bad started to stack up and take residency in your subconscious. This means that on some level, you actually started to believe that these messages were true.

And this is what happens even if you were lucky enough to have been brought up in a loving, emotionally supportive household. What about those of us who lived in families that were moderately to fully dysfunctional? The additional messages that were stored would be even more damaging to our self-esteem!

Our level of self-esteem determines what we will and won't accept from life. Our level of self-esteem determines what we think we are worth, from all perspectives. What we think we can earn, the type of people we associate with, the quality of our clothes, our cars, our houses, and so much more are all tied into our self-esteem. And so is our weight!

It just makes sense that if you hold yourself in high-esteem, you will treat yourself with respect and care. Conversely, if your self-esteem is low, your self-respect will be low too. Low self-respect does not translate into treating yourself well. Treating yourself well does not include habits that lead to an unhealthy body. And an overweight body is an unhealthy body.

This part of the program is going to work on changing the way you think about yourself, including learning to love yourself. And if love seems too strong a word, just work on liking yourself for now.

You have some unique talent(s) that others admire in you.

We need to go back to the subconscious, and offer it some new programming. As we've already discussed, the subconscious is affected in two ways....either by the constant repetition of an idea until it is finally stored, or through a huge emotional event that in an instant changes the way you think. For the purposes of this program, we are going to use the first method of reprogramming, constant repetition.

Do you know that you are a marvelous creation? A truly remarkable human being? That there is no one else on this planet who has the exact same make up as you? You are as unique as a snowflake! And did you also know that you have unique gifts to offer? Whether you are a great singer, dancer, crossword-doer, baker, parent, friend, artist, writer, sunset-watcher, gardener, decorator, cook, bowler, story-teller or anything else, you have within you the capacity for greatness! You have some unique talent(s) that others admire in you. Think about what this is. If you aren't sure, or if you can't even begin to believe you have such a talent, ask your nicest, closest friends for some insight. Your friends will be able to tell you what they see you being good at. We are going to use this information in just a minute.

No one is perfect, and we all have areas for improvement. However, we also all have areas of strength, and this is what we want to focus on, to celebrate. Years ago we were taught to focus on our weaknesses, and to work hard to bring these areas up to par with our strengths. And what did that really do? It created a nation of people all walking around feeling frustrated and bad about themselves, because they were focusing on the "bad" things about themselves.

Fortunately, now we know that there is a much more effective method for each of us to use to improve ourselves. All we have to do is know what we do well, and learn to do it even better! This has us focusing on our inherent strengths, on the things we naturally do fairly well and with ease. This helps us feel better about ourselves as we train our talents to become even stronger! In any area in life, what we focus on increases and expands. This is one of the natural laws of life. So it makes sense to focus on the good so it expands, and not waste energy on the negative, so it shrinks.

Now that you have identified what your strength(s), we are going to begin to reprogram the subconscious into understanding and believing that you are a good, lovable, worthy person! Think about how you would treat another person you thought of as being good, lovable and worthy. It would be very different from how you would treat someone you thought of as bad, unlovable, and not worthy, wouldn't it? Well the same is true for how you think about and treat yourself!

We are going to use the affirmation technique we learned in Chapter 4 of *Why Are You Weighting?* Just as a reminder, an affirmation is a statement you repeat over and over and over again to yourself, until you actually start to believe it because it is programmed into your subconscious. An affirmation is always done in the present tense, even though sometimes this can be quite a stretch of the truth! So, to make it easier for you to get going, we are going to start with your personal area of strength that you know is true. This way we can "shore up" your belief, and give you a good solid foundation.

A great way to start an affirmation is with the words "I am so happy and grateful now that I _____" and then fill in the blank with your strength. So you might say, "I am so happy and grateful now that I am a great gardener, with a beautiful garden of gorgeous flowers" or "I am so happy and grateful now that I am a great parent of a wonderful child" or "I am so happy and grateful now that I am a great singer/artist/seamstress/bowler/salesperson, etc."

Right now, I want to you to formulate your affirmation, and then memorize it. You are going to repeat this statement to yourself many, many times every day. You may want to put Post-it® notes all around to remind yourself to do this! I personally have affirmations on my bathroom mirror, in my bedroom, and sometimes even in the kitchen! You can't overdo this, and the more you do it, the faster your thinking will shift. Aim to say your affirmation (out loud or silently depending on where you are at the time) at least 100 times per day!

Again, don't be concerned if it feels as though are really exaggerating or even lying to yourself. Just keep repeating it over and over and over each day, and it will begin to feel like the truth because it will become the truth! The more your autopilot is bombarded with these ideas, the faster they will take root, and the faster your autopilot can get to work on making them reality!

You will soon begin to like yourself more and respect yourself more, which will begin to change your outlook on just about everything! You'll be amazed! Everything in your life will change for the better as a result of doing these affirmations over and over and over again. It really is a small price to pay for the incredible results you'll get!

The reason everything in your life changes for the better when you increase your self-esteem and self-respect is because doing this also changes the "lens" through which you look at the world. Each of us sees the outside world relative to our inside world. All our points of reference are internal. By changing internally, you are also changing your lens. So it is not really that the outside world has changed, it's just that you have changed how you look at it. You will begin to notice things you never noticed before, and won't notice things that used to get your attention. It's like looking through a telescope... you will see only what you focus on. By moving the telescope, your view will change. That doesn't mean the other view is not there, only that it is no longer in your line of sight. Changing the lens through which you look at the world will change what you see and what gets your attention. This is a guarantee!

An optimist sees the glass as half-full, and the pessimist sees the glass as half-empty. Did you ever stop to realize that they are both right? They are just looking through different lenses; the object they are looking at does not change at all. Both optimists and pessimists have very different ways of relating to the world, and as a result, the world reflects back their different views. This is how both groups can "prove" they are right!

Please decide right here and now to be an optimist about yourself (self-love) and your ability to reduce and/or maintain your ideal body weight. It doesn't matter what has happened before this moment. From now on, know you can do this. Love yourself, love your body, and just watch what happens!

Love puts us in a position of power, real power — power to change things both internally and externally. Love is positive, and it can move mountains. Remember, mountains can appear as other people, or even just as our self-talk. Begin today to treat yourself and talk to yourself in a loving manner, and you will begin to possess a special power that will change your world.

Just a note on love... Please remember, too, that most other people are walking around with the same (or even greater) feelings of self-doubt and unworthiness you had when we started this chapter. Begin today to treat all people as lovable and worthy even if it is obvious to you that they do not feel the same way about themselves. We can all use a little more love in our lives everyday, and by treating people, all people, with love and respect, you will be doing your part to improve the world everyday. You will be astounded by the difference in people's reactions to you when you approach everyone this way. And by loving others, you actually increase your self-love as well, because after all, we're all in this thing called life together, and on some level, we are all connected. Become an ambassador of good feelings, and share this message with others, even if it just through something as simple as a smile!

Chapter 6 Summary

- You are a magnificent being worthy of being loved!
- Those who think well of themselves treat themselves well.
- Affirmations are a very effective method of reprogramming our thoughts.
- Treat everyone you meet with a loving, respectful attitude.

Join with the other members of the www.WhyAreYouWeighting.com site as we all learn to love ourselves and each other!

_____

_____

_____

_____

_____

_____

Be not the slave of your own past. Plunge into the sublime seas, dive deep and swim far, so you shall come back with self-respect, with new power, with an advanced experience that shall explain and overlook the old.

Ralph Waldo Emerson,
(1803-1882) American Essayist.

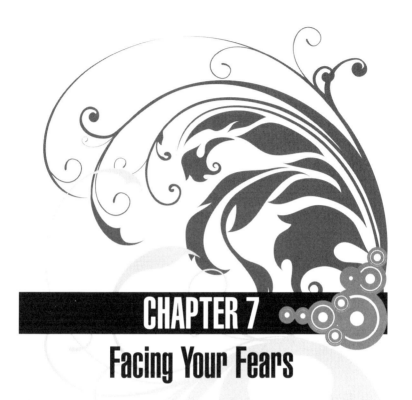

CHAPTER 7
Facing Your Fears

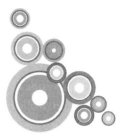

Chapter 7 - Facing Your Fears

IF YOU ARE ANYTHING like I was, you hate your excess weight, you don't understand why you keep regaining it back, and you berate yourself every time you gain a pound or eat a "bad" food. All this adds up to a lot of negative mental energy going on around your weight.

Have you ever thought about any positive aspects to your weight?

At first, this can seem preposterous! How can excess weight possibly have a positive side? Well, that's what we are going to find out in this section of *Why Are You Weighting?*

From the day we are born, as we move through life, we develop certain behaviours and attitudes to help us get what we want. For instance, we all learned pretty quickly that crying would get our empty stomachs filled or a wet diaper changed. That doing our chores would ensure we got our allowances. That studying for an exam got us better results. These are all fairly obvious, and it's easy to see the how the actions got our results. These are also pro-active, meaning we started the interplay, rather than reacting to someone else's actions. We wanted food or a dry diaper, so we cried. We wanted to have spending money, so we did our chores. We wanted a good mark on the exam, so we studied. These were all instigated by us, and motivated by what we wanted.

We also learned much more subtle methods, often without any conscious realization at all of what we were doing. This happened mostly in response to what was going on around us. These methods are known as "coping mechanisms," and we developed them in all areas of our lives. We all develop certain behavioural and thinking patterns in life as a method of responding, reacting, or just plain getting through specific situations. This process goes on our entire lives, not just in childhood. However, childhood coping methods (sometimes inappropriate ones, at that) can carry over into adulthood, often with out the the person being aware of what is happening.

The purpose of this section is to help you further understand why your body feels compelled to hang onto your extra weight by looking at what in your life you are "responding to" through your weight. In other words, to find out *Why Are You Weighting?*

And this is where you will have to put on your "sleuth cap" and really get to work to uncover the hidden agenda behind your weight. And I am here to help you do just that.

Don't worry if there is nothing immediately apparent. Your brain has done a really good job of keeping this info under wraps, and it will fight to keep it there. Your job is just to keep looking, to keep an open mind, and to finally uncover the hidden agenda so that you can understand it and adjust it.

Here is a small list of some of the reasons that people carry around extra weight:

To keep a partner
To avoid a partner
To get attention
To deflect attention
To avoid certain activities
To ensure certain activities

In other words, to protect themselves.

PROTECT THEMSELVES FROM WHAT? From what they fear. Fear is one of the strongest motivations for humans. Most people will work harder to avoid something they fear than they will work to get something they want. And this is where things get interesting because this is where they get personal — really personal.

The excess weight can act as a protector of sorts. It can be a buffer against whatever you fear, providing armor against the outside world. The physical body will always react to whatever thoughts are rattling around in the mind. In fact, Louise L. Hay wrote an excellent book called *"You Can Heal Your Life"* in which she teaches that all physical manifestations, whether disease, pain, or even bad skin, are related to something going on in your mind. In this book, Hay says that the probable cause of excess weight is "Fear, need for protection. Running away from feelings. Insecurity, self-rejection. Seeking fulfillment." She goes on to say that fat is related to "oversensitivity. Often represents fear and shows a need for protection. Fear may be a cover for hidden anger and a resistance to forgive."

Hay even gets specific about where on the body you store your fat. According to her book, fat in the arms can mean "anger at being denied love." Fat on the belly can mean "anger at being denied nourishment." And fat on the hips can be "lumps of stubborn anger at the parents." Even fat on the thighs can be "packed childhood anger, often rage at the father."

You can see that all of these are related to a thought or an emotion, in this case either fear or anger. All teachers of mind-related subjects will tell you that there are really only two pure emotions, fear and joy. All the other emotions are just different forms of these two. The positive emotions we experience, such as happiness, excitement, and love, are all just forms of joy. And the negative emotions, such as anger and frustration, are

All teachers of mind-related subjects will tell you that there are really only two pure emotions, fear and joy.

forms of fear. I think if you ponder this for a while, you will come to see that this is correct. The next time you find yourself angry or frustrated, spend some time thinking it through and seeing what it is you are really afraid of. It might be of not getting what you want, of being used, of being ripped-off, etc. This is actually a great way of finding out what is really going on at a deeper level when you do find yourself experiencing a negative emotion, and will help you work through the feeling so that you can get what you ultimately want. And this is true of everything in life, not just your weight.

We are all different, and what scares one person exhilarates another. Think of standing at the top of a snow-covered mountain. If you love skiing, this would be a really joyful moment for you. However, if you are scared of heights, this would be terrifying!

Only you can figure out why you keep the weight, and how it is protecting you and serving you against whatever it is you truly fear. We are now going to look deeper into ourselves to try to understand. Please remember that this is a process, and the time frame will differ for everyone. Some of you may have huge AHA! moments fairly quickly, and some of you may search for a long time before the answers come. There is no set amount of time this will take; everyone is different. Please commit to this process regardless of how long it takes. The results will be worth it, guaranteed!

I recommend that you dedicate some time everyday to working on this. Find a quiet spot where you won't be interrupted and really focus on this. It can be lying in bed first thing in the morning or just before you drop off at night. It can be at lunch as you take a stroll through a park. Or it can even be locking yourself up in the bathroom for five minutes of privacy! No matter where you choose to do this exercise, it is very important that you be kind to yourself, really kind. Occasionally things will come up that make you uncomfortable, sometimes very uncomfortable. However, carrying around your extra weight is uncomfortable, too, so this exercise will helped have to release all the discomfort, both mental and physical.

What I mean by being kind to yourself is not judging what you discover. You may have an AHA! that seems so obvious now, you will wonder how you ever missed it, and then that can lead to thoughts along the lines of "I have missed that? I am so stupid." Really listen to your "self-talk" as you go along through this, and when you catch yourself berating yourself (and you will; you are only human!), replace that thought with something more positive and self-loving. For instance, instead of thinking "How could I have missed that, what is wrong with me?" catch yourself thinking this, and then consciously say to yourself, "I am so grateful that I have made a discovery about my weight, and I am so happy now that I can find new, more effective ways of coping."

Everyone is different, and this is a really personal part of the process. There are no right and wrong answers here! This is really getting to know yourself on a level much deeper than you have probably ventured into before.

In my case, it took me a while to figure out that I was keeping my weight on because it was providing a buffer between me and the outside world. My weight was an armor of sorts, a protection from what scared me. In addition, it provided all sorts of great excuses when things didn't go my way, and allowed me to blame my failures on something other than myself.

For instance, if a date didn't go well, it had to have been because I was fat, not because I basically was an unhappy person. If I didn't get the job I wanted, it must have been because I was fat, not because I hadn't properly prepared for the interview. If someone snubbed me, if was because I was fat, not because I was giving off "leave me alone" vibes.

Being fat allowed me all kinds of excuses! The excuses increased my self-pity, and ultimately increased my sense that I was a victim in life. Anytime anything went wrong I asked myself "Why me?" and the answer always came back "Because you are fat."

So how was this serving me at the time? This "victim" way of thinking allowed me to continue on in life without having to take any responsibility for my results. It was easier for me to say that a date didn't call again because I was fat than it was for me to recognize that I probably wasn't a lot of fun to be around because I wasn't really a very happy person. It was definitely easier for me to blame not getting the job on my weight than it would have been to spend some time learning about the new company and its ways of doing things so that I was impressive as a job candidate. And to blame my weight as the reason people at social gatherings generally didn't talk to me certainly allowed me to ignore the fact that I was coming across as an aloof, unfriendly person...not exactly someone who others would want to initiate a conversation with!

So my weight became the crutch on which I leaned to avoid really looking at myself objectively. And to keep myself in denial. And to use as an excuse for staying unhappy.

It takes a certain amount of introspection coupled with courage to be able to stand back and say, "I didn't get called for a second date because I was incredibly needy and unhappy, not because I am fat." Or, "I didn't get the job because I was lazy about my interview preparation, not because I am fat." Or, "people at the party didn't initiate conversations with me because I stood in a corner like a wall flower, not because I was fat." In each case, I had to take responsibility for the results of my actions!

Earlier in this chapter I mentioned that weight can be a protector, to keep you away from what you fear. So let's look at some examples from my life about dating, jobs, and socializing from the perspective of fear and see how my weight was "protecting" me.

FEAR # 1: Being Abandoned. By staying fat, which I believed was preventing me from getting into a relationship, I was protecting myself from potentially being abandoned one day.

FEAR # 2: Not Being Good Enough. By staying fat, which I believed prevented me from getting a better job, I was protecting myself from the possibility that I might end up getting a job for which I feared I just wasn't good enough.

FEAR # 3: Not Being Likeable. By staying fat, which I believed was the reason people at social events didn't talk to me, I was protecting myself from the possibility that I just plain and simply wasn't likeable.

Please note that these three fears are all actually based on me not really liking myself. If I had liked or loved myself more and accepted myself, I would have most likely have assumed that others would like me, too. I wouldn't have immediately assumed that a relationship meant I would eventually be abandoned, or that I wasn't good enough to get the job, or that

I wasn't even likeable in a social way. My self-esteem was low, and so I expected to get bad results. Please go back and re-read the chapter on "Loving Yourself" if you are not sure about the point I am making here. This is an important concept.

It didn't happen overnight, but through journaling and introspection, I came to recognize the ideas I really held about myself. I feared I would be abandoned, so it was better to avoid a relationship in the first place. I feared I wasn't good enough to get the job, so it was better to mess up the interview than discover that I really wasn't good enough if I gave it my all. I feared that I wasn't likeable, so it was better to stand in a corner at parties, than to actually try and possibly fail at making friends and just confirm that no one liked me.

Much easier to blame it all on being fat. Much easier! So, my autopilot continued to help me remain fat by continuing to guide me into behaving a certain way (overeating) to get a certain result.

It wasn't until I found the courage to face my fears head-on that my autopilot began to realize that there was no longer any "purpose" to my fat, and started to release it. My autopilot then began to guide me through a different set of behaviours, such as eating normally.

On dates, I acted more confident and less needy. Was this hard? At first, yes. And did it result in being asked out a second time? Yes, it did. So was it worth the discomfort of changing a behaviour to get what I wanted? Yes, it was!

And once I realized that being in a relationship did not mean it had to end by being abandoned, my excess weight was no longer a reason to keep me out of a relationship. I no longer needed the weight to help me with this fear.

At job interviews, I took the time to do the research beforehand. Was this hard? At first, yes. And did it result in me getting a better job? Yes, it did. So was it worth the discomfort of changing a behaviour to get what I wanted? Yes, it was!

And once I realized that I did have what it took to be a good employee, my excess weight was no longer needed to protect me from being seen as not good enough. I no longer needed the weight to help me with this fear.

At parties, I forced myself to mingle with others, and not stand alone. Was this hard? At first, yes. And did it result in more people talking to me? Yes, it did. So was it worth the discomfort of changing a behaviour to get what I wanted? Yes, it was!

And once I realized that I was likeable, my excess weight was no longer needed to keep me as an outsider. I no longer needed the weight to help me with this fear.

It really is this simple. Not *easy* mind you, but simple.

Enough about me. Let's look at you and your situations. You are afraid of something, even if you don't think you are. You are human, meaning you have fear, probably of more than one thing. Remember, these discoveries will take some time, so don't rush through the process. Go slowly and appreciate every piece of data you find about yourself and your fears. It can be fascinating really getting to know yourself, to uncover what drives you to do what you do. Remember to be kind to yourself, and not judgmental. Just notice what comes up for you.

If you are not already doing so, you are going to begin today writing down your thoughts.

Keeping a journal or a diary is a great tool to help you figure all this out for yourself. Start by writing every day, even if it is just for 5 to 10 minutes. Don't censor yourself. Rather, keep your journal hidden away from prying eyes so that you can be completely honest in your writing because you don't have to worry that someone else might read it.

As you write, be sure to make note of your feelings that day. How did you feel when you woke up? At midday? After work? In the evening? How did you feel about yourself and your body? What challenges came up for you that day?

Note whether you had a day that moved you closer to your goals or one that moved you further away. In either case, pay attention to the details of the day. Did you wake up in a good mood or bad? Did your mood change during the course of the day? Who were you with? What did you talk about? What activities were you involved in? Then move into the less tangible aspects of the day, such as, "What were you thinking about?" What thoughts were you holding about yourself? Who or what were you afraid of? What makes you uncomfortable? When do you feel the need to overeat?

Look for patterns between what you are doing, who you are doing it with, how you feel, and what you are thinking. Look for these patterns in both the negative and the positive aspects of your day. These patterns are there; you just have to find them. Everyone's patterns are different, but we all have things that "trigger" us to think and behave in certain ways. Becoming aware of these patterns is the first step toward changing them.

Awareness and realization usually come along in small increments. Each day you may learn something new about yourself and how you cope with the world. And as this new knowledge begins to pile up, you will find yourself (your autopilot) naturally making changes in how you think, react and behave.

And then every once in a while you may have a huge realization that may rock you to your core. These types of realizations can cause a huge emotional reaction, which may take you some time to reconcile. And that is ok. Especially during these times, take care to be gentle and kind with yourself. Really watch your self-talk, and speak lovingly to yourself.

Whether your AHA moments are small or huge, you will have moments when you become emotional, so it is important to release that energy somehow. If you need to cry, by all means cry. Perhaps a walk around the block might help. Or grab a pillow and beat your fists into it. Find a way that works for you to release this energy, or it will turn inward and affect your autopilot in a negative way.

And as you discover things about yourself, don't beat yourself up! Please remember that you can't change the past, but you can change how it is affecting you today and tomorrow. Here's an example from my own life.

It took me a long time, a really long time, to realize that a friend named Cindy was a huge trigger for me. After spending time with Cindy, or after talking on the phone, I would unconsciously (thanks to my autopilot) move to the kitchen, open the fridge, and start eating whatever I could get my hands on. When I finally realized the relationship between my contact with Cindy and my mindless eating, at first I was really mad — mad at her for "causing me to do this," and mad at myself for allowing myself to do this!

Then I looked a little deeper, and realized I was really mad with Cindy on many levels, and that I was eating to stuff down the anger I was really feeling. I had done such a good job of stuffing the anger that I didn't even realize it was there. I was surprised at the level of anger I had found.

I was even more mad when I discovered this! Mad at the wasted energy! Mad at her! Mad at me! Really, really mad! And I had to face the anger, not eat around it. This meant I had to feel the anger, really feel it. And that scared me! I was so mixed up, moving back and forth from fear to anger and back again. For days I cried rivers of tears as I tried to figure out what all this meant now, and what it would mean for the future.

The first thing I realized was that I needed to break contact with Cindy for a while. So I did. I couldn't see how I could get over the anger when being in her presence made me angry.

Then I realized that I needed to forgive myself for not even knowing that I was angry! And once I recognized it, I began to see how my "invisible" anger was ultimately hurting no one but me. I have to tell you, this was hard. I had been beating up on myself for so long that it had become my "natural" way of thinking. (That's the autopilot again!) I began to see that my eating to avoid the anger was really hurting me.

And while I was working on releasing the anger, I had to find coping mechanisms other than eating. It is said that "Knowledge is Power" but I really believe it should be "Knowledge coupled with Action is Power." My realizations alone wouldn't change my weight. I had to take different actions to get results. And so I looked for new ways to express my feelings rather than eating around them. None of these steps I mention are easy things to do. And yet they are so worth doing, because now you can get to the root of the problem rather than just treat the symptoms.

> I had to find different coping mechanisms other than eating.

Going on a diet only treats the symptoms of excess weight. Until you dig down and discover the cause (fear, anger, etc.) you will never experience true "resolution" of your weight issues.

As I look back now, I can tell you that whatever short-term pain I dealt with in figuring all this out for myself was far less than the pain of living with my weight on a day-to-day basis.

And that short term pain was nothing compared to the joy of living life as a healthy-weight person! I would gladly do it all over again in an instant if I had to.

So, everyday be thankful for the small realizations that come to you. And when the big ones hit, and they will, don't use them as excuses to fall back into your old habits. Use the energy from these big emotions to fuel your journey to new levels of awareness, thinking, and behaviours. Work through the discomfort, pain, and fear, and come out the other side a stronger, healthier version of yourself!

A note here on working through emotions. Sometimes we can go it alone. Sometimes we need outside help to get us to where we want to be, and there is nothing wrong with that. A good counselor or therapist can help you see patterns that you may not be aware of, and offer up suggestions to make breaking these patterns easier. Be careful who you choose though to help you through this. Stay away from anyone who may have his or her own issues wrapped up in yours. Speak with someone completely objective. Perhaps a friend can recommend someone. Or ask your doctor or clergy-person for a name. Or go to the self-help section of your bookstore and look at all the titles! It is beyond the scope of this book to cover every possible emotional situation, and there is bound to be a book written by someone who has successfully navigated whatever you are going through.

The journey will all be worth it, I guarantee it!

Chapter 7 Summary

•   Childhood coping mechanisms can carry over into adult life.

•   Weight can be a protection from what we fear, and can be an excuse to avoid looking at what is really happening.

•   Journaling is a great tool to help you get to know and understand yourself better.

•   It's OK to ask for professional help to get you through an issue.

Please visit www.WhyAreYouWeighting.com to read about what others are doing as we face our fears together!

_____

_____

_____

_____

_____

"The mind's first step to self-awareness must be through the body."

– George Sheehan
(1918-1993) American Physician, Author and Running Enthusiast.

CHAPTER 8
Being Perfect

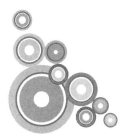

Chapter 8 — Being Perfect

AS I WAS WRITING this book, and starting to talk about what I was doing, people began to open up to me and share the tales of their weight journeys. And while everyone's story was different, I noticed that there was definitely a common theme, one of perfectionism. And so the idea for this chapter was born!

I am a "recovering perfectionist"! I say recovering because every day I work on letting go of my perfectionist tendencies. This is yet another example of how my thoughts are changing each and every day.

I have to admit I didn't know about the trend of perfectionism amongst those with weight issues. I certainly never thought of it about myself. No seminar ever pointed it out to me, no book ever talked about it, and no diet group ever discussed it. So since discovering this tendency in overweight people, I have spent a lot of time thinking about this, and I have a theory I'd like to share with you now.

For most of my life, I just thought I held myself to higher standards than others did. I never thought of myself as actually being a perfectionist. I believed that if something was worth doing, it was worth doing perfectly! (Note that this is not the same as doing something well.) I now realize that this was in order to receive praise from others, which then boosted my self-esteem.

I've tried hard my entire life to please. I've worked to please my parents, my teachers, my bosses, my friends, my dates, my landlords, my co-workers, even my grocery store clerk! Everyone but myself! If you were in my life, you could pretty much be assured that I would do whatever it took to please you. And in my mind, pleasing everyone meant being and doing everything perfectly.

I thought it was hard being perfect. What I didn't realize at the time that it is actually impossible to be perfect, so I persevered — perfectly, of course! Can you imagine the pressure I put on myself?

I always tried to look perfect, so I learned a lot about how to do hair and make up. Because I was so large, and there weren't any stylish clothes options for large people in those days, I sewed all my own trendy clothes — perfectly, of course. I guess my thought process then was that as long as I looked perfectly put-together, maybe people wouldn't notice that I was overweight. I now realize I was trying to hide the fact that I felt far less than perfect on the inside. I had almost no self-esteem, and what little I did have came from the glowing reports I would get after I had finished something perfectly.

And I did a lot perfectly!

I was the perfect student, bringing home straight As. This gave me the identity of being a great student, a real boost to my self-esteem. Until I got a B on something...and then I was a mess! I would berate myself for not having studied harder or longer, which of course then lowered my self-esteem even further.

> **I berated myself, again because I didn't have the self-esteem to recognize what was really happening here.**

I was the perfect employee, always doing what I was told, when I was told, and I received lots of accolades. Until I ended up having a boss who was very competitive and petty and who seemed to feel threatened by me. She gave me the worst job review of my life. This threw me into a tailspin where I blamed myself for everything that had happened, not realizing at the time that I was dealing with an immature, inexperienced boss. I berated myself, again because I didn't have the self-esteem to recognize what was really happening here.

I was the perfect friend. If you had a problem, no matter what time day or night, I would be there to help you out. This fed my self-esteem. However, if no one had a problem, there was no "food" for my ego, and my self-esteem would suffer. I also didn't treat friendship as a reciprocal event, meaning that when I had a problem, I felt that I couldn't discuss it with anyone, for fear of appearing less than perfect. Friendship is a two-way street. By insisting on being perceived as perfect,

I missed out on the great benefits of being able to share a problem of mine with a friend, and I robbed my friends of the chance to experience the giving side of friendship. And since I didn't share my troubles, they would seem to multiply in my mind, again lowering my self-esteem. (There is a saying that "Joy shared is joy doubled. Trouble shared is trouble halved." I now realize that this is so true!)

A comment here about self-esteem. It is not something someone else can give you (external). It is a gift you must give to yourself (internal). When you rely on outside forces for your self-esteem, you never know how things are going to go. You may be feeling great and then all it takes is one wrong look or word from someone else, and your self-esteem comes crashing down. True self-esteem is built from within, and can withstand the external forces that try to tear it down.

Perfectionism is really based in fear. Fear of being wrong, Fear of being criticized. Fear of losing control. Fear of being not good enough. On some level, I think we realize that we can't control everything that is going on around us. But we can control our own actions, so to allay all these fears, we strive to be perfect.

So now we add to the list of fears the fear that we may fail at being perfect! And fail we do because perfectionism doesn't work. We are humans, not robots, which means that we are inherently less than perfect. Remember the adage, "To err is human"?

So here is where I believe the weight issue enters the equation. Perfectionism is based in fear, and so is our weight. (Please see the chapter "Facing Your Fears" for review on how weight is related to fear.) Both are ineffective methods of dealing with fear, and we have already discussed many steps required to release the weight as you release the fear. Now let's look at releasing the perfectionist tendencies too!

I truly believe it is our flaws that actually make us interesting. Any hand made item is worth many times more than its mass-produced cousin because of the unique differences in the handiwork. Perfection is boring, plain and simple. People like non-perfectionists better than perfectionists. Our human flaws actually make us more likeable!

Mistakes are a great teachers! We learn from our mistakes. So if there were no mistakes, there would be no growth. As long as we learn from each mistake we make, and don't repeat the same ones over and over again, mistakes are good things. Think of a robot, a machine designed to do things perfectly each and every time. Once you got over the initial novelty of having a robot around, it would actually become pretty dull in its perfection. People are interesting, not robots!

How do you know if you are a perfectionist or simply someone who just likes to do well? Here are some points to ponder:

A perfectionist tends to focus only on the outcome, and not on the process. Non-perfectionists enjoy the journey that gets them to their goals.

Perfectionists set unattainable goals and then get frustrated and angry with themselves when the goals are not reached. They question their self-worth. Non-perfectionists set reasonable, attainable goals, and then congratulate themselves on reaching these goals. And even if the goal is not met, a non-perfectionists don't take it personally...their reactions generally relate only to the specific situation rather than their self-worth.

A perfectionist feels that what is accomplished is never quite good enough. A non-perfectionist is satisfied with the results.

A perfectionist will feel the need to give more than 100 percent to a project, or will feel like a failure or feel mediocre. A non-perfectionist will realize that there is only 100 percent available, and will work accordingly.

Interestingly, it is has now been proven that perfectionists ultimately end up attaining less than their non-perfectionist peers. Perfectionist attitudes interfere with success and rob people of the satisfaction from doing a job well. ("Well" is never good enough for a perfectionist.)

A perfectionist can get so caught up in the minute details of a project that the "big picture" is lost. This is why perfectionists also tend to be procrastinators. In the mind of a perfectionist, a project can't start until all the ducks are in a row, all the details figured out. This "paralysis by analysis" slows down the project, and often derails it altogether. This is why ultimately non-perfectionist will actually accomplish more.

Even relationships are affected by perfectionism. Often perfectionists will delay getting into relationships, because they are always searching for some "perfect" person who really doesn't exist. And perfectionists in relationships tend to hold their partners to the same unattainable standards that they hold themselves to, so of course the partners fail repeatedly to live up to these standards, causing friction.

I think I developed into a perfectionist for a number of reasons. First, I found school and learning incredibly easy, so to raise the bar for myself and make learning more interesting, I began to expect that I could do projects and write exams perfectly. I once spent a week being upset with myself because I only got a grade of 101 on a test when I could have gotten 102 because there was a bonus question. I even argued my point with the teacher. Looking back on this, I see that the teacher must have thought I was nuts! Perfectionism is a common trait in gifted students.

In addition, some of the people around me in my younger years were perfectionists, so in an effort to not let them down and to avoid their criticism, I strived for perfection so often that it became a habit.

In my own life I've had to build a new habit of non-perfectionism. My perfectionism was affecting my work and my relationships. (And also my weight, although I didn't realize the correlation until much later.) I can honestly say that giving up my expectations of perfection from myself and from others has led to a much more satisfying life professionally and personally. I still strive to do well in all that I do, but I have a more realistic idea of what doing well means. I definitely get more satisfaction this way, and enjoy the things I do a lot more than when I thought I had to do things perfectly!

Giving up perfectionism first requires an awareness that it is there in the first place. If you are not sure if you are a perfectionist or not, ask a couple of your close friends or associates. Trust me, they will know!

Then watch your reactions and self-talk. Every time you berate yourself for being less than perfect, train yourself to have a supportive reaction. I have learned to change my self-talk from, "Oh, you are so stupid!" to "I am intelligent. I just made a mistake." We forgive others for mistakes they make; we must allow ourselves the same grace!

Perfectionism is a habit and like all habits, requires concentrated effort to change. Don't expect that you will be a perfect non-perfectionist! Allow yourself some slack. Here is another area where affirmations can help. Form an affirmation such as "I am a human, by definition not perfect. Mistakes are a part of learning, so I am grateful for my mistakes and what they continue to teach me — I am not my mistakes, I am me — glorious, wonderful me, and I am a unique individual and unlike anyone else on the planet!" Memorize and repeat this affirmation whenever you find yourself falling back into perfectionist ways of thinking.

If you are really struggling with this, I recommend you get some professional help. Perfectionism is ultimately a destructive force to not only the perfectionists themselves but to the people around them as well. It is not a fun way to live, and can, in fact, steal the joy out of living. As a former perfectionist, I can tell you that life is much better now that I have learned to control this aspect of my thinking! And you can do the same. It will be worth it, I promise!

Chapter 8 Summary

- Perfectionism is a learned habit and, like all habits, can be changed.
- Perfectionism is a form of protection from what we fear, just as excess weight is.
- Perfectionists actually accomplish less in life than non-perfectionists.
- Perfectionism negatively affects your life in all aspects, both professional, and personal. It even affects your relationships.

Join us at www.WhyAreYouWeighting.com and become a member of our community where we are all working on being more human and less perfect!

_____

_____

_____

_____

_____

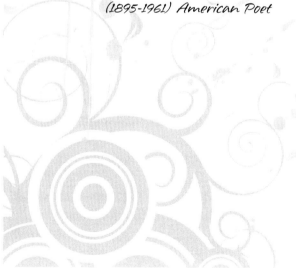

Perfectionism is a dangerous state of mind
n an imperfect world.

Robert Hillyer
(1895-1961) American Poet

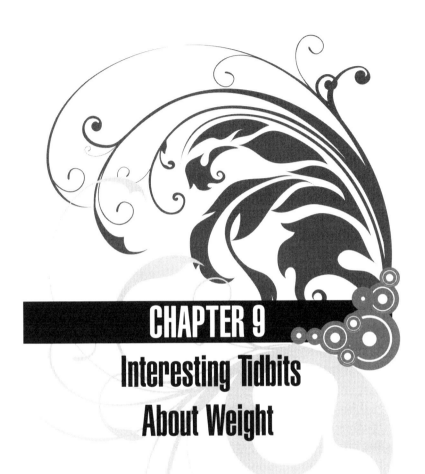

CHAPTER 9
Interesting Tidbits About Weight

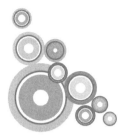

Chapter 9 – Interesting Tidbits About Weight

HOW OTHERS REACT WHEN
YOUR WEIGHT CHANGES

FOR ME, WATCHING HOW others have reacted when I finally achieved and stayed at my ideal weight has been a fascinating experience! I would never have thought that what I weighed had any real bearing on anyone else however, I know now that it did. Let's look at why.

One of the tendencies of human nature is to compare ourselves with others. Often we will compare ourselves with someone in a worse situation, to make our own seem better. And this does have some merit. For instance, it is hard to feel bad about yourself for getting in a fender-bender when a mile down the road you pass the scene of a fatal accident. This can help you put difficulties into perspective and keep you looking at the bigger picture and the more positive side of any situation. Using the car accident example, seeing the fatal scene would cause thoughts along the line of "Thank goodness I am still alive and the car just needs a wee bit of body work!"

However, remember that just as we are comparing ourselves to others, others are comparing themselves to us!

So this means that as your weight stabilizes and the new ideal-weight and ideal-thinking person in you emerges, you may notice some resistance from those around you because "things have changed." Specifically, how they see themselves in relation to you has changed. Most people do not like change, especially when the change is not their idea! And their paradigms or autopilots are going work really hard to keep their self-perceptions the same, and that can affect you if you are not aware of what is happening.

But it's your weight, not theirs. How can your weight affect them? Think of what has changed for those around you as your weight changed. Let's look at a couple of examples.

First, are any of your friends "food buddies"? People (of any weight) you know you can overeat around because they love food too and are never judgmental of your portion sizes? They may now be concerned that the friendship won't include food anymore, or if it does, that you might begin to judge them for their food choices. They aren't going to like this and may begin to consciously or unconsciously sabotage your weight-reduction/maintenance efforts.

Are any of your friends also overweight...but maybe not quite as overweight as you (were)? As your weight lightens, what changs for them is how they perceive themselves relative to your new weight. If you were always the "heavy one," it could now be that they fear being referred to as "the heavy ones"! And again, they aren't going to like this and may end up working to keep you as you were (heavy) to keep things the same for them. They most likely are not even aware that they are doing this.

Or you may have some friends who are even heavier than you were, and they thought of you and themselves as part of a a "club" where membership required extra weight. Together you could talk about the injustices done to heavy people, or go shopping at a large-sized store, or just sit around being comfortable (i.e., not feeling judged) in each others' presence. Basically, your new ideal-weight body means that you no longer belong to this club, and the other members will not be comfortable having you as part of it. They may try to sabotage your weight efforts, although probably not knowingly, to keep you part of the club. However, as you continue through life at your ideal weight, eventually you are not going to want to be part of this club as you no longer fit the criteria for membership. Unless these friends start down the path you are already on, you are better off without these people in your life. (I am not saying they are not nice people, just that for now at least, you are better off avoiding people who may have a stake in sabotaging your efforts.)

You may have a friend or associate who always has to be the centre of attention. Just imagine how that person may feel now that you are "stealing" some of the attention! As we all know, reducing your weight can draw a huge amount of attention. People will be asking you how you did it, and telling you how terrific you look. People who never paid you the time of day may now notice you. You will be wearing a new wardrobe, often with sexier pieces than you would have dared wear before. All this is going to draw attention to you for how healthy you are now looking and how well you are carrying yourself. Your attention-hungry friends may do all that they can to either reduce the attention you are getting or to draw it back to themselves. Either way, your weight has had an effect on their behaviour!

In each of these examples, your weight change has caused other people to have to take a look at what they are doing and who they are. And unless the timing is right and they are truly motivated to change as well, you will not be an inspiration to them, but rather a reminder of the things they have failed to do in their own life. They will naturally compare themselves to you and not like where they fit in the new scenario.

It's important here to remember that this is all happening on a subconscious level for those around you. They most likely aren't even thinking about this or actively working "against" you. However, just as our autopilots run us, their autopilots run them.

I believe this is why so many "well meaning" people really try to thwart your effort...because of the changes they are going to have to make to accommodate the new you! I am not saying this is conscious. I know most often it isn't. It is just their paradigms fighting to keep everything as it was. You're not the only one with a stubborn autopilot, that's for sure!

So be aware as you go out into the world in a new "re-packaged" version of yourself. This is going to have a ripple effect on those around you, and you need to know this.

Give those around you the time and space they need to adjust to the "new" you. In some cases you may have to give lots and lots of space, sometimes even permanent space. Some of my friendships have changed dramatically, in fact, even been lost, because that's what I had to do for me to stay on my new path. Eventually I found it too challenging to stay friends with people whose paradigms conflicted so strongly with my newly formed ones. After all, "birds of a feather flock together," and I had radically changed my feathers, so I found new birds to flock with!

PHYSICAL AND ENVIRONMENTAL FACTORS AFFECTING WEIGHT

FOR MANY YEARS IT was believed that only two things mattered with regard to weight control, food (input) and exercise (output). The thought was that as long as your output exceeded your input, all would be fine. To gain weight, increase the input or decrease the output, and visa versa for releasing weight.

And to *some* extent, this is true. However...

Rcently there have been some discoveries that are worth mentioning here as they may assist you in your efforts.

First, did you know that it is impossible to release weight if you are not sleeping properly? More on this in a minute.

Second, did you know that being dehydrated causes you to hold onto weight? And that you become dehydrated long before you become aware of the feeling of thirst in your mouth?

Third, if your body is malnourished, you will overeat because your body is screaming for nutrients. It is hard to believe that in our modern, developed society anyone could be malnourished, yet many people are.

Fourth, diets don't work. They cause weight-gain down the road.

Let's examine each of these further.

SLEEP. HOW IS IT CONNECTED TO WEIGHT?

It turns out that when you are in the deepest stages of sleep, called Delta sleep, many things are happening in your body. For instance, this is where most of the repair and rejuvenation in our bodies happens. Every day we go out and face the world, and life just causes our bodies to break down a little bit. Then when we go to sleep, when we get down into the deep levels, our bodies fix the little things that broke down that day, and we awaken feeling ready to face another day! This is really important, and is the reason why sleep quality (not just quantity) is the #1 determinant of health and longevity. Good sleep = good health.

Another thing that happens down in the Delta levels of sleep is hormone production and delivery. Many systems in our bodies are regulated through hormones, which are one method various parts of our bodies use to communicate with each other. For instance, it is the sex hormones that tell the reproductive organs it's time to get activated, which initiates puberty. Disruption with these hormones can cause an array of dysfunctions, from infertility to cancer.

After a meal, the hormone insulin tells our various cells to open up to accept the food that is awaiting delivery in the blood system. When this hormone is disrupted, diabetes or hypoglycemia may develop

And there are a couple of hormones (leptin and gherlin) released during the deep phase of sleep that are responsible for regulating appetite and metabolism. Metabolism is the rate at which your body burns calories. A person with a high metabolism can generally eat more food without gaining any weight, and may in fact have trouble keeping weight on, than someone with a lower metabolism, who may gain weight very easily.

Ideally, these two hormones work together to keep our body weight in check. However, just as with other parts of the body, things can go wrong with the hormones, causing problems to occur. In this case, the problems arise as body weight issues.

Leptin is responsible for dulling your appetite and for letting your brain know that your stomach has had enough food. It makes sense then that if your leptin levels are out of whack, the communication between your stomach and your brain is going to get disrupted. This can then lead to you overeat. If your brain doesn't not know when enough is enough, you will keep eating long after your stomach has been satisfied.

Gherlin is responsible for stimulating your appetite. Again, if the levels of gherlin are out of balance, your body is going to be sending some wrong information to your brain, indicating that you need food when really you don't.

So, it is of the utmost importance to ensure a good's night sleep. Here's a little Yes/No quiz to determine if you have a sleep challenge or not. (You may be surprised!)

- When I lie down I fall asleep the minute my head hits the pillow.

- I wake up one or more times during the night.

- When I wake up, I feel groggy.

- I work shift-work.

- In the afternoon I feel tired, sleepy, or have lower energy.

- I have to have a coffee first thing in the morning.

- During the night I toss and turn a lot.

- When I get out of bed in the morning my muscles are stiff and sore.

- When I get out of the bed in the morning I have limited range of motion.

- I hit the snooze button repeatedly.

- I snore heavily, and often wake myself up with a snort.

A "yes" answer to any of these is an indication that you may have a sleep challenge, and this could be one of the missing pieces as to why you haven't been able to properly maintain your weight.

I wish I had known all this years ago, as I was one of those kids who never slept, never! I remember being six years old and hiding under the covers at night with a flashlight and a book so I wouldn't get caught by my parents. I just couldn't sleep! And at the age of 6, I weighed 90 pounds! The average is 47 pounds. Then, as I matured into a teenager, my sleep deprivation continued, and I was 215 pounds when I was 15 years old. I had emotional issues around food, there is no doubt about that; however, I was grossly overweight, much more than my food intake alone should have caused. Every time I went to the doctor my thyroid would be checked, because they couldn't believe that I was getting that big given what I was (honestly) telling them I was eating. My thyroid was always fine; they never did find anything wrong with it.

I never slept through the whole night in my entire life! And this pattern continued well into adulthood for me, as did my pattern of yo-yo dieting. I never really had a problem reducing my weight once I put my mind to it. My problem was always keeping the weight off once the diet was over. I literally was either on a diet and reducing, or off a diet and gaining weight. There was no in-between. My non-dieting weight fluctuated by as much as 30 pounds in a month!

In fact, it wasn't until I was in my early 40s that I finally found a solution that worked for me, and for the first time ever, I got a good night's sleep. I awoke rested and refreshed and have continued to do so almost every morning since then. And I have to admit that maintaining my weight has never been easier than it is since I solved my sleep problem. I worked on my emotional issues, which certainly helped, and the sleep bit has definitely been the missing link for me. I encourage you to seek help if you are not sleeping, and in the chapter called "Recommended Resources" you will find references to what I found worked for me.

DEHYDRATION. HOW DOES WATER AFFECT WEIGHT?

TO EXPLAIN THIS, we need a mini-physiology lesson. Cells are the building blocks of our bodies. Cells make up tissues, and tissues make up organs, and organs make up our bodies...it all starts at the cellular level. So any process in our bodies starts with the cells. And just as it takes energy to get our whole bodies moving, it takes energy to get the cells moving! Cells get their energy from food or water. Sometimes they need food, sometimes they need water. Our bodies have ways of letting our brains know which it is, food or water, that we need.

However, modern eating habits have changed our bodies enough that our brains become confused sometimes by the signal and can't tell if it is water or food that is being required. This is known as getting the thirst and hunger mechanisms confused. Most often, it is the thirst signal that gets mixed up. The brain mistakenly assumes that the body is hungry and directs you to go get something to eat, even though it is water that was requested. Since this doesn't answer the initial request for more water, the cells send the signal again, only to have it misinterpreted once more, and the cycle continues.

You must be getting approximately 2 litres or 2 quarts of water a day to meet your body's requirements. This means water, not coffee, nor cola, not juice not milk. It must be water.

And not all water is created equal. Today we have myriad choice bottled, tap, filtered, reverse osmosis, and distilled are just some of the options. However, it is important for you to know that some waters act as water should, and some don't.

You are probably wondering what this mean. How should water "act"? I'll try to explain at least as far as the body is concerned. Again, it all comes down to what is happening in the cells of our bodies. Water, when it is "behaving" properly, is able to freely pass in and out of all our cells, fulfilling the cells' needs for energy. When the water is not behaving properly, this is not possible, and the cells start to suffer and problems of all sorts arise!

Modern-day water options, with very few exceptions, do not produce water that acts as water should! This is because the water has been heavily processed to make it safe from germs and bacteria. And so this water, while "safe" to drink, is really ineffective as a hydration source. These types of waters can cause health problems down the road because of this inability to do what water is supposed to do in our bodies! Even though you may be drinking the required amount, your body could still be in a state of dehydration because of the waters inability to adequately hydrate the cells. In fact, it is estimated that 75 percent of North Americans are dehydrated, despite spending millions, almost billions on bottled water. There is definitely a relationship between the type of water being consumed and hydration levels.

So be sure to really investigate various water treatment options when deciding which water to drink. In the chapter called "Recommended Resources" you will find references to what worked for me.

MALNOURISHMENT. HOW IS IT POSSIBLE TO BE OVERWEIGHT AND YET UNDERNOURISHED?

AH, THE PARADOX OF our modern times! There are two factors to consider when looking at food. First, the amount of calories being consumed, and second, the amount of nutrients being consumed. There can often be a big disparity between the two.

Modern-day food, for the most part, is heavily processed. We rarely get a food item direct from its s source. Most often it has had some type of processing done to it first. This processing varies from food type to food type, it suffices to say that unless you are buying directly from the farmer your food has almost certainly been processed in some way to maintain freshness and shelf-appeal during the long transport from the field to the store. The upside to all this is that we are able to buy local, domestic, and even exotic imported food products out-of-season that all look great! However, the downside is that many of the nutrients, vitamins and minerals that were initially in the food get sacrificed along the way.

The same thing applies exponentially to fast food. Fast food is fast because something has been done to it to allow it to cook more rapidly or more easily, or to last longer, or to even taste better. Again though, all these "improvements" actually diminish the nutritional value of the food. And with fast food, extra fat has often been added to increase the pleasure factor in your mouth. (Fat is the reason chocolate feels better in your mouth than celery!)

So let's look at calories versus nutrients. You may be trying to eat a daily allotment of food that falls within your calorie guidelines for your height and weight. However, your food may not contain all the nutrients your body needs, so your cells will signal to the brain that more food is needed. Your brain will then tell you to eat, although if you are continuing to feed your body nutrient-deprived foods, your body will continue to be undernourished, and the cycle continues, eventually resulting in weight gain. It is not the vitamins and minerals that cause you to gain weight; it is the calories, plain and simple.

The answer these days is to supplement your food with vitamins and minerals to ensure that you are meeting your body's daily requirements, regardless of the types of foods you eat in any given day. I believe that everyone needs to be supplementing, regardless of whether you eat organic or fast-food. We all need it!

A comment here on supplements. They are not all created equal, both in pricing as well as in format. Please see the chapter called "Recommended Resources" for references to what I found worked for me.

DIETS DON'T WORK. HERE'S WHY.

THERE ARE A COUPLE of factors that result in why diets don't work. One is physiological (the body) and one is psychological (the mind). Let's look at both, starting with the body.

I mentioned metabolism earlier, and said that it is the rate at which your body burns calories. There is a measurement known as your BMR, or Base Metabolic Rate, and this is how many calories your body needs at its resting rate to perform its life-supporting duties such as keeping your heart beating, your lungs working, your blood circulating, and your brain thinking. This does not include exercise or any other activities. The higher (or faster) your BMR, the more calories your body requires to support itself.

Everyone's BMR is personal, and it is hard to change. However, there are a couple of ways to affect it, either to slow it down or to speed it up. When you are looking at weight reduction or maintenance, you are going to want to speed it up whenever possible. Exercise speeds up your BMR, and the effects last for up to 16 hours post-activity. Building more muscle on your body is the only way I know of to increase your BMR permanently...permanent as long as you continue to have the muscles! This is why exercise is such a great complement to any type of weight-management program. It makes it easier!

Low-calorie diets, on the other hand, do just the opposite. The body has a great capacity for adjusting to its circumstances, and when the body is left long-term on a low-calorie diet, it goes into "starvation mode" in order to ensure its survival. This starvation mode includes lowering (slowing down) your BMR, to ensure that the minimal calories coming in everyday are enough to support your vital organs. This slowing down, though, seems to be come a long-lasting adjustment. So it follows that when you stop dieting and begin to eat normally again, your body now needs fewer calories than before, so your normal amount of food in fact becomes too much, and the body stores the excess as fat. It is very hard to reset your BMR once it has been lowered. Exercise helps, but it seems that once you have a lowered BMR, you may always have a lower BMR.

This is the reason why so many people who go on low-calorie diets end up gaining it all, and often more, back when they go off the diet. These are the physiological reasons behind why diets don't work.

Now let's look at the psychological or emotional reasons why diets don't work. It all comes down to deprivation. A low-calorie diet is hard mentally, especially in modern times. Everywhere we look there are ads for food, really great looking food. Most of our social events include food, and just about every celebration there is revolves around food. We are a society obsessed with food! And when you are on a long-term calorie-restricted diet, if you are sticking with it, you are going to start feeling deprived sooner or later. It is just human nature. And once the feelings of deprivation kick in, you can kiss your willpower good-bye! No one is strong enough mentally to be able to continue to be self-deprived forever when it comes to food. Feeding ourselves is primal; it is required for survival. The body has very strong mechanisms around food, and it can override just about any conscious decision when you are hungry. You may only fall off the wagon for a brief time, like a meal or a vacation, or maybe even fall off permanently, and then what? If you are like most of us, you will start to berate yourself for not being strong enough, for not having enough willpower, and that sends your self-esteem plummeting, which can cause you to then want to eat for emotional reasons. Low-calorie diets are just not a good idea, and should be avoided if you are serious about getting control of your weight.

And one last note on this. By now in this book, you have no doubt come to understand the idea that your thoughts can cause your feelings. And if you are thinking about how deprived you are, that is not going to cause a good feeling to happen in your body. If you stay focused on the deprivation, you are going to crack, because you are only human!

So what should you do? Ideally, find a food plan (notice I didn't say diet!) that allows for flexibility, and lets you find a way to enjoy your favourite foods on occasion. If, for instance, chocolate is something that you can't live without, then don't!

Find a way to balance your food choices so that you can have some chocolate. (Or ice cream, or cookies, or what-ever your fave foods are). If you deprive yourself altogether of your favourite foods, you are going to become obsessed with them, and then sooner or later, your brain will grow tired of being obsessed and drive you to get some of your forbidden food, in spite of your willpower. Then you start to berate yourself.... See where this leads? Nowhere good, I can tell you! Nowhere good.

Your weight-releasing efforts should never result in any reduction more than 2 pounds each week. If your weight is releasing at a quicker rate than that, you are in danger of lowering your BMR, which, as discussed, has long-term side effects. Monitor your food intake until you can easily release 1 to 2 pounds per week. This level will allow you to enjoy a wide variety of food, including your favourites, and will prevent your brain from taking over and causing you to fail! And while this 2-pound rate may seem a bit slow if you are looking for a quick fix, it will really help you easily maintain your weight once you are done. Weight that comes off quickly goes back on just as quickly. So go slow, and enjoy the process. Learn to enjoy your food, and to eat slowly. Your body will thank you and work with you, instead of fighting you every step of the way!

Chapter 9 Summary

- Others will react to your weight changes as they compare themselves to the new you.
- Sleep, hydration, and nutrition all play a role in the physiology of weight.
- Exercise raises your BMR, while a very low-calorie food plan lowers it.
- Avoid deprivation with any food plan; include some of your fave foods to stay satisfied.

Join our membership at www.WhyAreYouWeighting.com and learn more!

_____

_____

_____

_____

_____

_____

"Most men pursue pleasure with such breathless haste that they hurry past it."

– Soren Kierkegaard
(1813-1855) Danish Philosopher

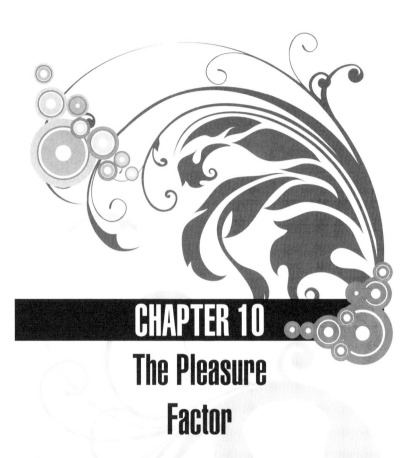

CHAPTER 10
The Pleasure
Factor

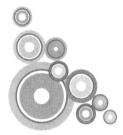

Chapter 10 – The Pleasure Factor

MY GOOD FRIEND DEBRA JOY is a wonder to be around. She is one of those special people who embraces life and lives with gusto! In fact, her professional life now is dedicated to helping others rediscover the joys of pleasurable living through her work with a program she developed and calls The Primal Bliss. I asked Deb to contribute a chapter to this book because I think she has some valuable words to share. So the rest of this chapter has been penned by Deb. Enjoy!

PLEASURES AND ADDICTIONS

LET'S GET SOMETHING CLEAR — Addiction is not pleasure. I know addiction is a big bad word, but we are a society riddled with addictions, so let's just deal with it. I speak from experience. I have an addictive personality. Like Mae West I've believed that too much of a good thing is wonderful. The most subtle and pervasive addiction I've dealt with is my addiction to sugar, which I will discuss later. I've also been addicted to work and the high I get from pushing myself to achieve goals. We can be addicted to alcohol, drugs, sex, shopping, work, food – you name it. All of these things can be pleasurable, but if you use any of them excessively, especially as a way to distract yourself from issues in your life, then it is most likely an addiction that you need to address.

Since addictions can feel good for a time, and since they can give us a rush we don't get from other places, how do we tell the difference between addiction and pleasure? Addictions feel good when we are indulging in them, but leave us depleted afterwards. They seem to be giving to us but they are in fact taking from us. When the high of the addiction wears off we feel tired, down, and sad, even resentful, shameful and guilty. True pleasures nourish us. After indulging in them we feel nurtured, expansive, joyful, peaceful, and good about ourselves.

YOU WERE MADE FOR PLEASURE

YOU ARE DESIGNED FOR pleasure. It is your birthright. Deep within you there is overwhelming happiness and joy. You might even call it ecstasy. Don't believe me? Let's consider your senses. They exist not just to help you survive this life, but to give you sensual satisfaction. The beauty of a sunset, the touch of a feather on your neck, the sound of a baby laughing, the smell of your lover's skin, the taste of rich chocolate melting in your mouth... none of these is necessary for your survival, but substitute each of those with your own favorite experience and you know your senses are capable of giving you great pleasure.

There's a reason we call children "bundles of joy." If you've forgotten the joy you felt as a child, just watch some kids for a while, and unless someone is making them suppress their joy, you'll see how often they express it. Pleasure is an incredible source of energy for kids. They wake up to a snow-storm and spontaneously jump for joy, clap hands, and feel excited to play in the soft stuff. Kids will play for hours as long as it's pleasurable. When the pleasure stops, they don't want to play anymore. It's that simple. Pleasure is their guide.

SO WHERE HAS YOUR PLEASURE GONE?

PERHAPS YOUR EXPRESSIVENESS WAS too much for one of your parents, or any adult in your life, and someone told you to "behave," "keep it down," or "grow up." All of those messages told you that your expression of pleasure was too much, or your tears of sadness were inappropriate, so being a good child you kept it down, "stuffing" down the joy. If you do see kids playing today you will see how excited they get, how they scream with delight. And then watch: before long you are likely to witness an adult telling them to keep it down, and being "good children" they probably will. I'm not saying that children should be allowed to go wild whenever they want. There is a difference between raising children to fit in society with respect for others and stifling their expression continually. Since this isn't a chapter on how to raise kids, I'll leave that for now.

It's not just your expressions of joy and pleasure that got stuffed down. As a child you may have learned to suppress your sorrow, disappointment, and hurts. Parents hate to see their children cry and often discourage it. In doing so, kids learn that they please their parents when they are "happy." You may have held your breath and tightened your belly to hold back tears.

This tightening of muscles becomes a habit over the years and creates an armor in your body, around your heart, your throat, and your belly. At first it feels protective. You don't get in trouble when you can hold your emotions in. You make your parents happy. But over time this armoring is the cause of dullness in the body and the psyche. It creates a disconnect between your body and your mind. When you become armored, you are no longer able to connect fully with the natural ecstatic feelings that wash through your body. Even orgasms will lack their full satisfaction.

In our society we want all of the "good" feelings without any of the "bad" feelings. We want love without fear, joy without sorrow, ecstasy without despair, and happiness without anger... but they are two sides of the same coin. If you won't allow yourself to feel the depths of your sorrow you'll never know the height of your joy. If you can't let yourself feel the clenching of your fear you can never feel the expanse of your love. We tend to hide these "bad" feelings away, hide them in the dark where they become part of our shadow. The shadow parts of ourselves are those parts we deny. Sometimes they go so deep into our subconscious that we are not aware of their existence at all. But even when we are not aware of them, they can still quietly rule our lives without us even knowing it.

In my family I didn't witness healthy expressions of anger. My dad had a terrible temper and would blow up, especially when he was drinking. Though he never hit us, I thought he was going to kill us one day. I walked on eggshells whenever he was around. Though I'm sure others in my family had lots to be angry about, I never saw anyone else expressing anger.

Since I never learned how to express it, I lost touch with my own feelings of anger. I lived most of my life not feeling angry about things that should have enraged me. Anger became so deeply embedded in my subconscious that I couldn't access it. Nature is always seeking a balance; Yin needs Yang. Light needs Dark. Not surprisingly, then, I always ended up in relationships with men who were very angry. Some had terrible tempers that scared me as my father's. That's one of the ways "shadow" feelings can rule your life. If you are not willing to acknowledge them and integrate them into who you are, you may either act them out in surprising and often unhealthy ways or you will keep attracting those characteristics in your partner, friends, and boss.

If you accept these feelings as part of your experience of life, if you will integrate them into who you really are, they lose their power over you. We tend to deny the feelings of anger, jealousy, fear, and shame, because somewhere along the way we were taught that those feelings are bad. Really feelings are neither good nor bad. They are just energy wanting to move through your body. It's what you do with them that matters. There are healthy ways to express anger, hurt, and sorrow. If you will allow yourself to express all of your feelings you will find that life becomes much more pleasurable for you, and probably for those around you too. I find if I will allow myself full expression of what I'm feeling, even if I don't know the reason for the feeling, I find a great deal of joy and exuberant energy just on the other side of the "bad" feeling. Sometimes I feel agitated, angry, and uptight without knowing why. I could try to be nice, and deny the feelings, but that doesn't really make them go away, and I waste a lot of energy holding those feelings in. The best thing I can do is to release those feelings to make room for new ones to come in. If I take a few moments and bash a tennis racquet on the bed, letting myself yell so that I am breathing deeply, it doesn't take long to exhaust those feelings and find myself feeling happy again, open to the pleasures life has to give me.

Try an experiment for a moment. Take in a really deep breath. Hold it. Don't let it go until I say so. (Don't worry; it will only be a few seconds in all.) Now take in a little bit more. Keep it in. Hold onto it. Is it starting to become uncomfortable? Are you noticing that all of your attention is now focused on holding it in? Are you starting to feel agitated that you have to hold it in? Are you noticing that there is no room for any other feeling?

OK – LET IT GO!

PHEW. DOESN'T THAT FEEL better? And you probably noticed that as soon as you let all that old air out, fresh air came rushing into your lungs without you even trying.

That's what it's like to hold in feelings that need to be expressed. If you want to suppress your anger and hold it in, or not bother anyone with it, that takes a lot of energy. It becomes uncomfortable for you, and it takes up room that would otherwise be filled with something new that wants to come in. Since it's not as life-threatening as taking your next breath of air, it doesn't occupy your mind as much as this exercise did, but you get the idea. Letting it go can feel so good! And that's what you want, right? To feel good?

HOW TO KEEP PLEASURE AWAY.

WE LEARN VERY YOUNG that some feelings are good and some feelings are bad. I remember experiencing many years of painful sadness as a teenager. My wellmeaning mom would say, "What do you have to feel sad about? You're smart, attractive, you have lots of friends...." When she'd ask that, then I also I felt guilty for being sad. "She's right," I'd think to myself. "I have a mom who loves me, a wonderful brother, friends, food and shelter. I'm being pathetic." The fact that I was having an existential crisis at 16, that I longed for a deeper connection with God and didn't know how to find it, didn't seem like good enough reasons to be sad. When I felt sad and despondent I didn't know any healthy ways to nurture myself. I felt guilty for being down when my life was so good. I didn't know it was ok to feel blue and really get to the core of my sadness. I didn't understand then that if I let myself really explore my feelings, and really express them, they would lose their power over me. Instead I stuffed the feelings with cookies, cakes, anything sweet.

In my family love was often expressed with sugar. My mom was the Queen of Fun, the Kool-Aid mom of the neighborhood. She was filled with energy, and sweets were given as expressions of fun and love. (We had chocolate cake for breakfast in our house!) My mom traveled a lot for her job and I missed her terribly when she was gone. I connected sugar with love and particularly with my mom, so eating the treats she had made or bought was a way of feeling her love. As long as I was chewing them I was distracted from my sadness, but the moment I stopped stuffing my mouth the sorrow was there, only now it was compounded with a sense of shame for having eaten all kinds of junk food. You can see what a vicious circle this was. I was so out of touch with my body in my teens that the only way I knew to stop eating was when I would reach the point of feeling sick. This never became an obvious problem to me or others because I never became obese.

Years of therapy of different sorts helped me face the pain I had felt in life, and over the years I learned healthy ways to express my anger and sadness. Once I integrated those feelings into my self-expression they no longer rule my life in subtle and sneaky ways. But I am still a work in progress. Recently I had an incredible weekend with my husband. Lots of laughter, love-making, deep conversations, playing in the ocean as dolphins swam by, and dancing. It was like a montage from a romance movie. After the weekend I found myself gorging on sugary cookies. I ate so much I felt exhausted. Sugar has that effect on me. Then I felt guilt and shame. "I know better," I told myself with disgust. After letting go of the shame and self-abuse, and instead becoming curious about why I would do such a thing, I realized I had maxed out on the pleasure I would allow myself — or as my friend says, "I had hit my head on the fun ceiling." My subconscious mind wanted to make sure I stayed within my own self-imposed limits, and an easy way to bring myself down emotionally and physically was to eat sugar. That was a huge AHA, moment for me. I realized there was nothing to be ashamed of. I had just reached my limit. The lesson for me was that I had to find gentle ways to expand my limit. Pleasure is like a muscle. You couldn't go from curling 10 pounds one day to 100 pounds the next-without your body responding in pain. I just needed to work my pleasure muscle some more.

WHAT WOULD PLEASURE DO FOR YOU?

HAVING MORE PLEASURE IN your life is absolutely going to help you with your weight issues. It's natural to want to feel full, especially for women. Women are biologically designed to be filled. Female bodies are meant to be filled when having sex, wombs become full when pregnant, and women (and men) want to have a life that is full. But this longing can become pathological and can lead to addictions. Rather than finding healthy ways to fill ourselves we become workaholics, shopaholics, and overeaters, stuffing ourselves to feel full.

If you were able to tap into the pleasure that is always present in your body, you would feel full without the need for external stimuli. The only thing between you and your natural ecstatic state is your ability to feel it. With very little effort you can learn techniques to help melt the armor around your body that separates you from your deepest feelings, and open the channels to bliss that are inside you.

This isn't about giving up foods, or going on a diet. In fact you'll find that you even get more pleasure out of eating, without the guilt, shame and regret.

HOW DO YOU BRING PLEASURE BACK IN?

WHILE THIS CHAPTER WON'T allow me to develop a specific program for you, here are a few important exercises you can do to bring more pleasure into your life. They each take only a few minutes, though you can do them for longer if as you like. (My contact info is listed at the end of this chapter if you would like more information on personal consultations and personalized programs.)

PELVIC BREATHING.

DEEP BREATHING IS ONE of the easiest ways to start to melt that armor in your body and to feel the feelings from which you have been cut off. Many people find that breathing deeply can often bring up feelings of sadness and anger, even when they weren't feeling those before the breathing exercise. If you are able to ride the wave of emotion that may come up for you doing this exercise you will find there is real pleasure in this breathing. It will become a treat you can give yourself at any time of the day.

THE EXERCISE:

LIE ON YOUR BACK ON the floor or a bed. With your legs parallel, bend your knees, keeping the soles of your feet on the floor. Relax your arms at your sides. Close your eyes and just breathe comfortably for a minute. Just notice your breath without changing anything.

Now that you are aware of your breath, inhale all the way down to your genitals. (Your breath won't really reach your genitals, but bringing your attention there will open up the diaphragm and deepen your breathing dramatically.) Exhale fully. Keep your belly soft. Continue this for a few minutes.

Now as you inhale arch your back slightly so you feel your butt press against the floor. Inhale all the way into your genitals. If you breathe slowly enough you will feel the oxygen filling you up like a glass of water. Starting in your pelvis, it moves slowly up your body to your collar-bone. As you exhale, relax your back on the floor, and bring a slight upward tilt to the pelvis. Be sure to keep your belly relaxed while doing this. As you exhale, you may start to feel the oxygen leaving your body from your collar-bone to your pelvis.

Continue to breathe like this for a few moments. Keeping your eyes closed, feel your breath like a tide coming in, filling your body as you inhale and arch your back, and going out as you exhale. Find the pace that enables you to feel like you are riding this wave. It's a sensation of surfing your own body.

This is an exercise you can do any time you feel stressed. You can do it while you are still in bed, if you want to start your day by getting connected to your body in a way that is easy and sensual. I do this when I feel an overwhelming craving for sugar. Pelvic breathing makes the craving go away, and brings me back into my body. I feel calm and centered and full again.

PELVIC BREATHING – SITTING.

SITTING IN A CHAIR OR cross-legged on the floor do the same breathing as above. Before you start the breathing make sure you really feel a connection between your "root" and the surface you are sitting on. To do this, tighten your anus, your genitals and your perineum (that's the space between your genitals and anus). You should feel your body rise up off the surface. Now, with an exhale, relax your anus, genitals, and perineum completely so you feel as though they are touching the floor or chair. This will make the breathing more effective.

Inhale all the way into your genitals; arch your back slightly as you feel the wave of oxygen move up your body. Exhale completely as you round back slightly and tilt the pelvis forward. Feel the wave move down your body.

To be effective these do not have to be big movements. They can be incredibly subtle. I do this when I'm driving, sitting on a bus, in a stressful meeting, or out for dinner and feel sugar cravings coming on. No one knows I'm doing it and yet it slows me down, makes me more aware of what's really going on in my body, and instantly brings me into a deeper state of pleasure.

EATING FOR PLEASURE

I RECOMMEND YOU DO this exercise once a day... just for the pleasure it will bring you.

I love food. I love eating and I'm good at it. I eat a lot. When my in-laws met me for the first time they all said, "She's a good eater!" I'm not overweight. At 5'4 I weigh somewhere between 110 and 115. I haven't owned a scale since I lived at my mom's house so I don't know exactly. But I do find eating to be a pleasurable thing to do.

I'll admit not all meals are enjoyable, and many are ordinary and simply done out of necessity, but whenever possible I like to bring as much pleasure as possible into eating.

For me the key to enjoying what I'm eating is to bring my awareness to it. That's not always easy. If you are like me you probably find that you are rarely just eating. You are eating and socializing, eating and watching TV, eating and driving, eating and reading, eating and walking, and so on.

THE EXERCISE:

- Take a piece of food that you enjoy and are about to eat. Let's assume it's chocolate.
- Take a good look at it, as though you've never seen it before.
- Examine the colour of the chocolate.
- Now really look at the texture, the nooks and crannies, and the size of it.
- Pick it up and smell it. How does the smell make you feel?
- Lick your lips. Run the chocolate along your lips. What does it taste like?
- Now put it in your mouth but don't bite it.
- How does it feel on your tongue? Against your teeth or cheeks?
- What does it taste like now that it's in your mouth?
- Now take a bite but don't swallow it.
- Is the flavour more intense when you bite it? Do you notice any flavour that wasn't there before?
- Smile. Does this change the flavour at all?
- Think of someone else who would enjoy this. How does that affect what you taste?
- Swallow. How does it feel in your throat?
- What is the feeling that's felt behind in your mouth? How long does it last?

This little exercise will take just a few minutes a day and can change your whole relationship to food. It enables you to get more out of the food you eat instead of eating more food.

My wish for you is that you will find more and more of life's pleasures are present all the time in your own body. You have everything you need to have a full and rich experience of life. You only have one life – enjoy it.

ABOUT DEBRA JOY:

JOY IS THE FOUNDER of The Primal Bliss, a movement-based therapy that releases physical and emotional blocks held in the body, enabling people to reconnect with their natural ecstatic state. She has a Masters in Leadership and Training, is a certified yoga instructor, and has practiced Tantra for many years. She coaches individuals to bring more presence and pleasure to their careers, relationships, and everyday experiences of life. To find out more about private sessions, classes or upcoming retreats go to www.ThePrimalBliss.com

Chapter 10 Summary

- Addictions are not pleasure.
- Pleasure is your birth-right.
- Somewhere in life you cut yourself off from your own pleasure, and you can reconnect to it.
- Experiencing more pleasure in your life would make you feel more full and satisfied.
- Some simple exercises can keep you in your body and away from temptations.

_____

_____

_____

_____

_____

_____

_____

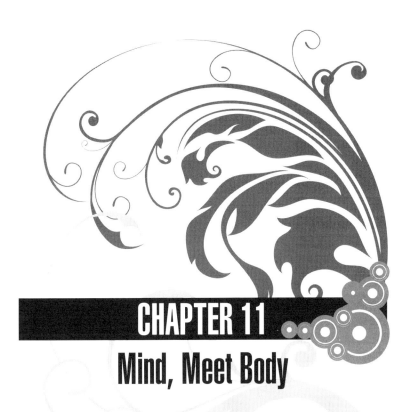

CHAPTER 11
Mind, Meet Body

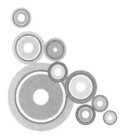

Chapter 11 — Mind, Meet Body

DR. NIMET MEGHJI AND her husband, David Lord, who are a dynamic couple in the Health and Wellness Field, wrote this chapter. I find their approach unique and effective, in that they address body, mind, and spirit in all that they do. I consider myself fortunate to be a client of their wonderful wellness clinic, called The Optimal Health Centre. I asked them to contribute a chapter because of their holistic approach and knew that they would provide some interesting angles on our topic, which they did! Enjoy!

It is usually easy for us to listen to the words or to read the facial expressions of others, but are you aware of what your own body is saying to you? Are you aware of what your body is feeling right now? Most of us are not in the habit of sitting and having a conversation with ourselves, even though it may be a good idea to do so considering we are with ourselves all the time! Ultimately, if we ignore our body it will eventually get very upset and really start talking. And if we still don't listen, it will start screaming! And at this point, we will have to listen, because if we don't then the cause of our suffering will continue. Please realize that it may take a while to understand what the body is trying to communicate, because we are not used to having a conversation with ourselves. It may even be awkward at the beginning, just as falling in love can be, but with time it will become more comfortable. In this chapter, we are going to look at how to use the wonderful ability that our body has to express itself to better understand our total selves.

On the macro level, our modern lives have weakened our connection with nature. We are living in a society that continues to overuse its resources on earth and pollute its water. The elements of earth and water are very important to the production of food. Bringing this to the micro level, the same is happening when the body starts gaining weight; the connection with the body and mind is weakened. Therefore, we are slowly removing ourselves from nature, we are creating barriers in listening to ourselves. Sometimes this barrier can take the form of fat. The more we are bombarded with non-natural stimuli, the more difficult it becomes to hearing our internal voice. If this internal voice really wants to be heard then the body gets bigger to take its place and competes with the distractions of the mind. Now we must take this opportunity to reintroduce each other. Mind, meet Body. Let's start with "Hello. My Body would like to get to know my Mind." A great way to initiate this is with an *Awareness moment.*

AWARENESS MOMENT

IN ORDER TO UNDERSTAND ourselves, we need to be aware. This will be the most important concept, this one of awareness. Let us practice awareness for a moment by doing the following:

- Find a comfortable position to sit or lay down.
- Focus on your breath first exhale from your nostrils and then focus on inhaling breath through your nostrils.
- Try to take breaths in through the nostrils and out through the nostrils. Just be aware of the breath without regulating it.
- Close your eyes, be still and observe yourself.
- Just observe and be aware of any sensations and thoughts.
- Accept these sensations and thoughts.
- Say a kind word at the end of your awareness moment.

Congratulations! You have taken a great step in connecting with yourself even if your awareness moment may have only lasted a few seconds. You can do this as many times as you like. Slowly work on this so that you do it for at least twenty minutes in the morning and twenty minutes in the evening. Awareness of oneself is a wonderful state to be in. Try to remember to observe and be aware of your sensations as you read this book. Over time, awareness will help you to choose the actions that are beneficial for you.

KNOWING YOUR BODY

AYURVEDIC MEDICINE IS A gift from India, dating back to 1500 BCE It is a complete form of medicine focusing on the cause of health problems by examining not just the body but the mind and spirit as well. The observation and the deep understanding of self by Rishis, who were dedicated to doing this, founded this art and science. Let us work with the wisdom of Ayurvedic principles to better understand ourselves, which will evoke an inner wisdom within us, bringing balance in our body-mind state. This in turn will bring balance to the spirit.

According to Ayurvedic principles, the body takes its form from five elements: water, earth, fire, sky, and air. Our individual constitution takes form from these elements. The three constitutions (or doshas) are Vata, Pitta, and Kapha or air, fire, and water, respectively. We are usually a combination of all three constitutions but we exhibit dominance in one or two of them. For example, one could be Kapha-Pitta, where Kapha is dominant and Pitta is secondary. During our lifetime, there may be variations as to which dosha is showing its dominance, but if we are in balance the constitution inherent to us will be in its natural state.

The following descriptions are a brief overview of the different doshas so that we can understand our body. The list is not complete and is only for the purpose of getting a general idea of the concepts. The characteristics listed may not all apply but we tend to exhibit clusters of these, and that would give us an indication of what doshas are dominant at any given time. Once we balance our body-mind state, then the presentation of the doshas is likely to change to reflect our true nature.

A Vata constitution would exhibit qualities of sky and air. These are some of the characteristics we may observe with Vata's body: The frame may be very short or tall, thin and narrow, and gains weight in the midriff. Under stress, Vatas are likely to lose weight, get constipated, or have excess gas. When their constitution is in balance, they are introspective, disciplined, perceptive, and spiritual.

Someone with a Pitta constitution would have the fire element. The body frame would be medium built, athletic, with a moderate weight. Pittas gain weight evenly. Under stress, they are likely to get ulcers, develop either gluttony, or undergo weight reduction. Stressed Pittas often exhibit insomnia, addiction to intoxicants, and diarrhea, and they love hot spices. When they are in balance, they are adaptable, intelligent, bright, and successful.

The Kapha dosha has the element of Water and Earth. These body frames can exhibit the characteristics of being heavy, strong, overweight, and they tend to gain weight in the chest, arms, buttocks, and thighs. Under stress there can be a tendency to oversleep or overeat, or a loss of appetite; Kaphas can also be anorexic or bulimic, tend to retain water, have lots of attachment to things, and tend to laziness. When their Kapha dosha is in a balanced state, Kashas are calm, contemplative, nurturing, and maternal.

If our body has excessive weight then the water and earth elements are dysfunctional, or our tendency is leaning towards being very Kapha. There is also Pitta or Vata present in varying degrees. We will focus on Kapha, as it is the common dominant dosha associated with significant weight gain. This may not be your natural tendency but challenging events in life may have made this attribute dominant and out of balance, which then would cause you to exhibit excessive weight gain.

In its natural state, Kapha's energy is there to sustain everyone as it contains the earth and water elements and thus is associated with Mother Earth. Its spiritual nature falls within the first and second chakras (body energy centres), which are the pelvic plexus and the genital areas of the body. The Kapha dosha keeps the family and home together, it is maternal. Kaphas provide nurturing to family and friends just as the earth takes care of us. Their nature is wonderfully calm and so both Pitta and Vatta gravitate to them, looking for this nurturing. They have grace, calm, and sensuality. The challenging work for Kapha, try, to detach from many of their cravings. They have to be aware of what they really need and what is excess. Being aware of this and working on it will keep them in balance.

Many of us face challenges in life but for Kapha personalities, there is a tendency to turn inward during times of difficulty. They may be depressed and will tend to keep things inside. This is dangerous. Instead of being the ones who build and keep things together, they become the destroyers. They may deceive others about who they are so as to protect themselves. A Kapha's senses of taste and smell are dominant, and under stress these qualities are amplified, which can lead to excess of food or even possessions.

To bring balance to the earth and water elements, a fairly strict daily schedule. They need to work on constantly being aware of their inner conflicts and to bring them out. Just as water needs to move, so do these doshas in order to keep healthy. Kaphas make good partners and exhibit stamina and nurturing.

A great day for a Kapha starts early in the morning with a shower, followed by meditation and yoga or a physical workout. Ideal breakfast time is from 8 to 9 a.m., and would include tea and a light but filling meal. Lunch would be at 1 p.m. and should be the biggest meal of the day, and then ideally the Kapha would go for a quick walk. A light snack should be taken at 4 p.m. so as to maintain an even pace during the day. A light dinner would be taken at 6 p.m. the Kapha if the meal is heavy at this time, lethargy will set in. Kaphas should sleep at least eight hours a night and some may want a bit more. Once we start becoming aware of what our body needs, then we are likely to make healthier choices.

KNOWING YOUR MIND

BEING AWARE OF OUR minds is just as important as being aware of our bodies. Practicing awareness moments is a great way to get a better understanding of ourselves. This will bring us to the present moment, which is a great start toward shaping our future. Our reactions of the past have shaped what is happening now, therefore we need to also look at these to shed light on the patterns we have adopted to cope. You may have encountered many difficult moments in your life that have left their mark and are still creating their effects. We will address past traumas to understand what happened to our state of mind. We have provided an awareness chart for you to fill in. It is important that you not ignore this chart, as you will need it for the analysis, which will follow.

TO DO NOW:

FILL IN THE AWARENESS Chart below. You may want to do this in a special journal book dedicated to this journey you are taking. Try to list five events that have made a significant impact on you. You can list more if you like as this is only a guideline. You may want to take an awareness moment before you start and anytime during.

THE AWARENESS CHART

List of emotional traumas you had in your life.	Year it happened	Your initial feelings to the trauma	Your behavioural reaction to the trauma	Your feelings today about it
(E.g.) Sexual abuse by relative	1981	Confused and Angry!	Started smoking and eating more	Less Angry Sad and sometimes Depressed
1)				

2)				
3)				
4)				

Try to be specific about your feelings and list as many tramas that apply. This may be difficult, but stay dedicated to it until you finish the chart. You may not finish it in one seating. Keep coming back to it until you have at least five examples. This is an insight into you. Take your time and be as clear as you can.

By filling in the awareness chart, you have already started an incredible healing journey. Even if you just have one example so far, it is a wonderful start. This is the type of effort you will need in order to make the desired changes.

Refer to your chart and see when you first started gaining weight. What was going on in your life? Did any weight correlate with a particular type of emotion you were feeling? During our early childhood years, the ego is shaping and is reliant on guardians to protect it. These are fragile years for the development of self as we give an implicit trust to those caring for us. Throughout our lives, an interdependency exists among us so the potential to feel hurt exists. When our trust is broken or not fulfilled, we can spend a lifetime reacting to it. What has happened so far and your reaction to it has made you who you are today. You need to be aware of this.

The reaction of eating to the point of gaining excessive weight has several interpretations. Perhaps you started hiding within this extra weight as a way to hide your feelings. Today may be the first time you realize that your eating was a way to push your feelings and emotions down so you wouldn't feel so much. As time passed, your emotions were suppressed by your weight so you could not really be in touch with yourself. Slowly this reaction turn into a habit and you found yourself automatically reacting to events in your life by turning to food.

Think about today and how you are feeling. Are your feelings connected with how your body is expressing itself physically? To a great degree, this is probably the case. Being aware of this connection helps you to understand yourself. As we get a better idea of who we are and our inner conflicts, there comes an understanding of our reactions to life. These reactions are what we have to work with to bring a deeper change within. Once we are aware that we are reacting, and understand what we are reacting to, we can bring real change.

Once you realize that the connection between your weight changes and those of your emotional state, awareness has been established. The time that you started putting on weight could have been a protection reaction. You may have been in a relationship where you felt you were not able to take your place emotionally or psychologically so your body tried to express this by taking on more weight. — For example, perhaps the person you were in a relationship with was aggressive, degrading, or manipulative, making it difficult for you to express your needs. Over time, this harm your self-esteem. The place that you were not able to take emotionally now translates into taking place physically. There is now a sense of isolation because you are not able to express yourself, and you are withdrawing inward for comfort. When we hurt, we try to protect ourselves. One way is to have a barrier of fat between our inner and outer world.

We could have experienced a situation in life that left us with a sense of anger and abandonment. In a situation of rape or abuse, the encountered trauma is often suppressed, as we do not want to remember it. We may rebel against people or situations out of anger from what has happened to us. This wall of anger provides a distraction to not look at ourselves as it is difficult to deal with what has happened. Anger then provides a great distraction from examining our feelings of abandonment because memories seem too painful. We struggle with the weight as we try to comfort ourselves with food.

You may have lost a loved one and are experiencing an emotional shock from the feeling of grief. There may be feelings of guilt due to the loss of someone near to us. This emptiness becomes hard to handle, which leaves us with feelings of abandonment. These events have left an aching emptiness that you are trying to be satiate by eating. This of course only starts a cycle of weight gain that works to alienate us further.

If our childhood years bore internal fruits of insecurity due to a lack of emotional or material support, then we may have begun to gather food to compensate for these unfulfilled needs. If we turned to food to fill this void then it could have been that we lacked the emotional support from the provider of food (most often this is our mother).

If you have been hypersensitive about your qualities and physical appearance, your body may be expressing this. The weight gain is to show yourself that you have been very critical and hard on yourself. As a child and even as an adult, you start rejecting yourself. Your thought patterns make small imperfections become much bigger, making it difficult to appreciate your positive qualities and physical appearance. The attention is put on what does not appeal to you, and the extra focus dedicated to this, results in the body putting on extra weight.

You may have a tendency to feel you need to keep many things. You may be holding insecurities and exhibiting fear of being exposed and vulnerable. You want to avoid being hurt by criticism or uncomfortable situations. All these conflicts are kept within and they accumulate. This gathering of thoughts and emotions will also make your body react the same way – to gather and store the food within.

There may be a feeling that you have limitations in some aspect of your life and that there is something you have not been able to accomplish. This feeling of limitation translates to the body expanding and becoming overweight so as to try and take its place. If you have been looking for a goal to accomplish in your life and have had difficulty with words and action, you may be trying to compensate with the physical body.

Our minds react when our bodies feel pain. If we are not happy with an event in our lives, our tendency is to have an aversion to the event and try to get rid of it. This aversion is so emotionally charged that our reaction to it is not necessarily based on what is good for our body and mind. The choices we make to resolve this hurt we are feeling at the moment is to suppress it or "deaden it." One way is to eat in excess beyond what our body needs because we are now trying to fulfill it emotionally rather then just physically. The association of food to feeling "better" in a major crisis has been made. The association of eating excessively as a means to protect ourselves physically and emotionally from the hurt may also be created. The repetitive reaction of eating excessively creates an attachment that becomes a defining part of our ego. Over time our image of how we define ourselves changes because of these reactions and their outcomes.

Our reaction of eating becomes so comfortable that we are not even aware that we are eating in excess of what we need. Because we are hurting inside, we may not care if the food we eat is harmful or beneficial. Over time, this makes us less aware of how a food reacts in our body so we may be ingesting harmful foods without realizing it.

KNOWING OUR ENVIRONMENT

THE OTHER FACTOR TO be aware of is the food we receive from our environment. Not knowing the damaging effects of some foods can cause problems. The public is not always made aware of the harmful effects of ingredients in processed foods. This can be very dangerous to our overall health as some of these ingredients can cause cellular damage. And, of course, if we are eating these foods in excess, then the damage is amplified. A simple guideline to keep in mind is that if Mother Nature created it then it is probably beneficial in moderation. We can learn about this from reading about nutrition or seek guidance from professionals. I highly encourage you to be informed about the food you are taking in. The essence of our being is nourished by the food we take in, so make sure you know what you are putting into your body.

Conscious awareness needs to be present when preparing your meal and when eating it. When you are preparing your food, if you feel stressed or agitated, take five minutes of silence by sitting in a comfortable place and focus on the breath going in through your nose, and out through your nose. In other words, take time for an awareness moment. To create an ambience, you can burn dried sage and play gentle music. You may even want to shut down the electrical appliances during your meal-times so the air will be buzzing with fewer waves. This will help to air out energies that you do not want transferred to your food.

Before you start each and every meal or snack, say some peaceful and loving words. This thought process will help the digestion of your meal.

BODY-MIND FAST

CHOOSE ONE DAY OUT of the week to do a Body-Mind fast. On this day, fast for 4 or 5 hours before going to bed in the evening. This means you will refrain from ingesting anything except water (water is also the only thing you should be having in the evening and the hours before going to bed). You may have as much water as you like. If this is very difficult at the beginning then have one fruit during this time. This is fasting for your body. You may be saying, "How can my mind fast, when all it does is crave for all sorts of food? What kind of mind fast is this?" At the beginning, yes your mind will be craving when it does not get what it wants. The mind will fantasize about eating at the first chance it gets. This is a perfect chance for you to observe your mind. Every time you think of eating, be aware of it and focus on your breath. Accept the thoughts you are having and focus on the breath. You can sit down or pause for a moment and observe your breath. This is your only job – to accept and focus on your breath going in through the nose and out through the nose. Practice awareness moments.

At the beginning of this practice, the mind will often think about eating, as this is its pattern. You may be surprised at how often your mind pattern is focused on food. Eventually, with awareness and acceptance of your thoughts and breath, this habitual pattern will change. You will find you can accomplish this with ease. Keep up this practice at least once a week as it allows the body to focus on regenerating itself rather then digesting when it rests for the night. This is very important for your body to heal. The next morning you will feel lighter. Over time, you may want to practice this a few more evenings or keep most evening meals lighter then your other meals.

HEALING

WHEN ONE BECOMES AWARE of how inner conflicts are manifesting in the body, the journey to healing has started. Imagery or visualization of what you want can bring you closer to your goals. If you can imagine it then you can achieve it. Imagine yourself with the body image you want. Create images that have an emotional charge. This will strengthen the association of your Self with the image. You can reinforce it by cutting out pictures that resemble your image and putting it in your bathroom and elsewhere so you can see them everyday. Looking at the eventual images of what you will be, and mentally reinforcing this image everyday, can be a powerful tool if done repetitively.

Dieting and exercise are tools that can be used to shed the weight but if you do not know the real source of the excessive weight it will be difficult to maintain your ideal weight. In other words, you must ask yourselves *Why Are You Weighting?* Initially the introspective search may seem difficult, but be diligent and the rewards will be exponential! Recognize the excess of emotions within. Accept them just as they are and then let them be. Forgive your guardians, who tried the best they could given what they knew. Understand that it really was the best they could do at the time. Start recognizing your value and all your possibilities. Start filling the inner emptiness with love and a positive feeling of yourself.

Start surrounding yourself with love.

Be confident in life and yourself.

Express emotions freely.

Ask the universe to help you. You do not have to be alone in this. Each day, ask the universe, God or nature to help you. Get a holistic or complementary practitioner, tell them what your goal is, and ask for help. Be diligent and conscious about your goals to shed the weight.

The focus is to bring balance and not be chasing after an illusion of perfection. The chasing can waste your essence of energy, for what we perceive as imperfection is actually an opportunity to be more conscious of ourselves. We can use our situation to work on ourselves, to really look at what is going on inside of our body and mind. Our awareness of the present moment will stop the reaction we are used to creating. This alone can bring profound beneficial changes.

ABOUT THE AUTHORS OF THIS CHAPTER:

Dr. Nimet Meghji, DC, HBA, CASCI

DR. MEGHJI PRACTICES BODY-MIND medicine with great success. Her studies in psychology, chiropractic, acupuncture, and Ayurvedic and Eastern medicine have helped her develop unique and effective combinations of body-mind treatments for her patients. Her practice is greatly influenced by Buddhist principles and meditation. Dr. Meghji is the mother of beautiful twin girls, aged 20 months, and with awareness is constantly learning from them. Along with her husband, David Lord, they operate the successful "Optimum Health Centre," a multidisciplinary clinic focusing on complementary medicine, in a beautiful, calm, Eastern-inspired setting. The mandate of the clinic is to provide and educate people with the art of balancing body, mind and spirit.

David Lord, Spec.Ed

DAVID LORD PRACTICES PSYCHOTHERAPY with a focus on understanding the spiritual self. His academic studies have been in the area of specialized education counseling. Lord embraced spirituality at a very young age with the support of his mother, who has been a pillar of love and compassion for him. His father contributed through teaching discipline and perseverance. Lord practice of therapy focuses on Buddhist principles, and his passion to discover spirituality in different cultures led him to travel China, Latin America, the United

States, France, Cambodia, Laos, Thailand, and India. Theses experiences strengthened his understanding of the mind and its characteristics. He loves his family, and finds that his best spiritual teachers are his wife and twin girls. David works to understand the true essence of happiness by focusing on meditation and spiritual research.

Both Dr Nimet Meghji and David Lord can be reached through their website at www.OptimumHealthCentre.com or at 416-913-3700.

REFERENCES USED FOR THIS CHAPTER:

Le Grand Dictionnaire des Malaises et des Maladies, Jacques Martel. Quebec City, Canada: Les Editions Atma Internationales, 1998.

Ayurveda, A Life of Balance, Maya Tiwari. Rochester, NY, U.S.: Healing Arts Press, 1995.

Prakrti, The Integral Vision, Volume 1-5. General Editor: Kapila Vatsyayan, New Delhi, India: Indira Gandhi National Centre for the Arts, L1995.

Chapter 11 Summary

- Practice awareness moments and keep an Awareness chart.
- Get to know both your body and your mind.
- Practice body-mind Fasting.
- Express Emotions Freely.

_____

_____

_____

_____

_____

_____

_____

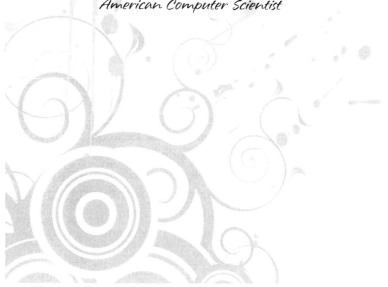

"The best way to predict the future is to invent it."

— Alan Kay
American Computer Scientist

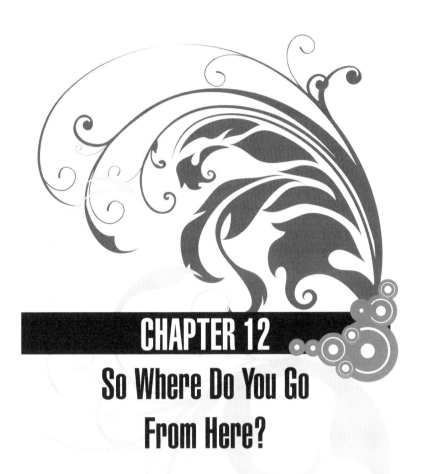

CHAPTER 12
So Where Do You Go From Here?

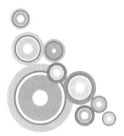

Chapter 12 – So Where Do You Go From Here?

CONGRATULATIONS ON MAKING IT through *Why Are You Weighting?* It is my hope that you are now beginning to look at yourself through kinder, more loving eyes, and really appreciating the marvelous creature that you are! I also hope that you have begun to recognize some of the patterns and habits at play in your life, and have begun to change or shift those that may in fact be moving you in the wrong direction.

Change of any sort can be uncomfortable! However, remember that it is only when we challenge ourselves, and when we move out of our comfort zones, that real change can begin. If we keep doing what we've always been doing, we'll keep getting the same results we've always had. We simply must change ourselves in order to get the results in our lives to change.

Now, you don't need to feel that you've got to do this alone! We have a number of options for you.

I invite you to join our free *Why Are You Weighting?* e-newsletter service. You will receive e-newsletters in your inbox that will be full of tips, reminders, and inspiration to keep you on course!

If you'd like to feel even more connected to others who are on a similar path to yours, then please go one step further and join our *Why Are You Weighting?* Million Pound Club. This is a group of people all committed to nurturing their new habits and helping each other stay on track with their new ways of thinking, as we work together to release and/or maintain a combined one million pounds of excess weight!

You can sign up for our e-newsletters and join our Million Pound Club at www.WhyAreYouWeighting.com. This site is a fabulous resource for all, and I encourage you to use it fully.

And I can't wait to meet you in person soon, at one of our *Why Are You Weighting?* Group Seminars. Please check the www.WhyAreYouWeighting.com website to see when we are coming to your area! And if we aren't scheduled in your area soon, why not become a *Why Are You Weighting* Area Coordinator to make it happen faster? Area Coordinators work together with us to put on local events. The satisfaction that comes out of knowing you are making the world a better place by sharing this information is unsurpassed. Please visit our website to learn more.

It has been my honour to share what I've learned with you, and I just know that all the information in this book will work for you just as it has for me! So don't delay! Get working on your affirmations today. Get a pen and paper and start journalling! Begin today to change the way you think about yourself and your weight. This is your life, no one else's, and no one else can do this for you. There will no doubt be moments that will be challenging; however, I promise you, promise you, that if you just stick with this, do the exercises and journalling, and continue to change the way you think, your life and your weight will both change for the better.

And at some point in the not-too-distant future, you will find yourself wondering "What was I weighting for?" as a great, big smile passes across your face!

Also, please let your friends, family, and acquaintances know about this book and the *Why Are You Weighting?* Program. The diet industry is not doing our society any good, and I am working to change all that, one person at a time. I know a lot of people, but I don't know everyone. I need your help to get this message out. Please help me get this info into the hands of those who need it. It is my long-term vision that every overweight person on the planet will become aware of *Why Are You Weighting?* and what it can do.

And please join our Million Pound Club at www.WhyAreYouWeighting.com. It doesn't matter whether you are at the start of your weight-reduction journey, and *Why Are You Weighting?* is helping you get slimmer, or whether you are already at your ideal weight as you discover the *Why Are You Weighting?* method of successfully staying there. Every pound that is not carried around as body fat as a result of this program qualifies to be entered into the Million Pound Club! Whether your story consists of 5 pounds of weight or 500, there is a place in the club for you! Please join me on my mission, and let's help people the world over discover the joys of being ideal-weighted forever!

Send me an email and let me know how you enjoyed this book and the concepts presented here. Please share your success stories with me. Keep in touch, and let's change the world together! Because now that you know *Why You Are Weighting?* it's time to let others know too!

Chapter 12 Summary

- We must change if we want to get our results in life to change.
- Don't do this alone. Join others on similar journeys at www.WhyAreYouWeighting.com site for support.
- You can become an Area Coordinator to bring *Why Are You Weighting?* to your area.

Be sure to join www.WhyAreYouWeighting.com
today and see all the tools and support we have available
to ensure your success!

_____

_____

_____

_____

_____

_____

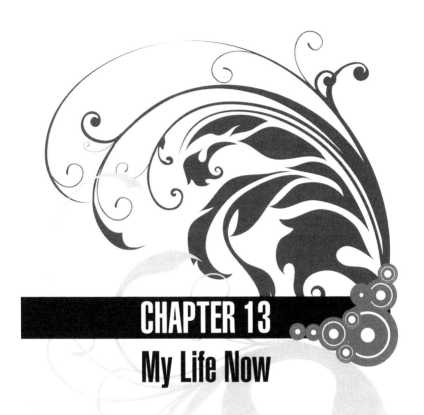

CHAPTER 13
My Life Now

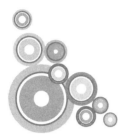

Chapter 13 — My Life Now

SO HERE WE ARE now nearing the end of this book. As I was writing this, a friend suggested that I do a chapter on where my life is now, and I thought that was a great idea. So here we go!

My life now is so different from where it was before I began my own *Why Are You Weighting?* journey that in some ways, my former life seems like a dream. (Or should I say a nightmare!) Today, I look at myself and the world differently, I think differently, I act differently, and I am a completely different person. When I look back at the person I once was, I have to shake my head to believe I have come from there to here.

You have read all about my "there" throughout this book, so now let's look at my "here," my current life.

I am more confident than I have ever been. If you had asked me to write a book back when I weighed 300 pounds, I never would have agreed, because I wouldn't have believed I had anything to say that would be of interest to others. I didn't believe I had anything to contribute. I had very little self-esteem and very little confidence in myself. Perhaps the greatest gift I've received through the process of growing and changing to reduce my weight is this new-found belief in myself! I am at the stage of my life where I now know that I can do anything I set my mind to.

This confidence has spilled over into many areas of my life. I am married to a wonderful man named Andrew. Instead of my old habit of sabotaging my relationships before they even had a chance (to avoid rejection), I gained the confidence necessary to venture forth into the area of love. Love requires vulnerability, and to be truly vulnerable requires being strong first. This new strength of mine is also related to my increased self-confidence. Andrew and I share a great life together where we are constantly growing and challenging ourselves professionally and personally. I think we have a great partnership, and I am grateful having him in my life. By learning to love myself, I opened myself up to loving others.

My friendships have definitely changed. Some of the friends I had back in my fat-days are now longer my friends, for many reasons. I was connected to some of these people through our common bond of being fat, so when I began to live as an ideal-weighted person, our bonds were broken. Some of these people have done little or no personal growth work over the years, while I have done so much that there is little or nothing we have in common anymore. I also realized that a lot of the people in my life back then were quite negative in their attitudes, so when I turned my attitude around, we just didn't click anymore. In fact, I think we made each other uncomfortable, so these friendships just faded away.

Some of my long-term friendships have endured and blossomed. It turns out there were many people in my world who saw things in me that I wasn't seeing in myself. And once I began to explore what I had to offer, these same friends offered me reams and reams of encouragement to keep me headed in the right direction.

I have also gained some remarkable new friends in the last few years. People who are encouraging, supportive and positive. People who "think outside the box" and help me do the same. People who lift and inspire me to be the best I can possibly be. These new friends are just some of the many blessings I have received as a result of changing the way I think about myself and my weight.

I wish I could say that I never think about my weight anymore, but that would be a lie! Every day I still have some weight-related thought; many of these are my old paradigms still trying to hang on by a thread. However, whenever I have any of these old thoughts, I now can recognize them for what they are, and basically just dismiss them or replace them with something more positive.

The hardest lesson for me has been accepting my physical body. I still have insecurities about my body, although they are significantly less than years ago. I just remind myself that even supermodels have body insecurities, and this helps me...in fact, I like knowing that I have something in common with super-models! The "old me" had a lot of shame about my physical appearance, which caused me to want to run and hide. The "new me" knows that everyone is different, and that everyone has physical assets. I now dress to highlight my assets, and this helps me feel more beautiful and confident.

I have learned to dress in styles that flatter my body shape and style. Not everyone can successfully wear every style. Find a style that works for you and stick with it. Wear clothes that make you look and feel great and update your look through accessories. I can now go out the door thinking to myself, "Stacey, you look great!" and then graciously accept all the compliments that come my way. Dressing well, in a style that suits my body type, is a real confidence-booster. If you are not sure about what your style is or should be, consult a good friend or even a professional wardrobe consultant who will give you honest feed-back and get you going in the right direction.

One of things that held me back when I was first thinking of writing this book is that I had not achieved a state of perfection with my weight. (There's that perfectionist thing again!) As long as I follow my own advice, everything is always great with my weight. However, I'm human, and I've had moments where I have lost sight of what I have learned, and I've temporarily "fallen off the correct-thinking wagon" so to speak. When this has happened, my weight has gone up and my self-esteem has fallen again. Or was it that my self-esteem fell, and then the weight began showing up again? I actually think the latter is more like it.

The biggest difference for me now though is that I can pick myself up much sooner and get back on the wagon of correct thinking long before the weight really starts to pile up. I don't beat myself up over it anymore. It just is what it is. And I remind myself that success in any endeavour is "the progressive realization of a worthy goal or ideal." (Earl Nightingale) As long as I continue to progress I am a success. It doesn't matter how many times I fall, as long as I can get back up again. And here's a paradox: The more often you get back up, the less often you end up falling. So if you do find yourself slipping into old habits, don't focus on what is going wrong, but rather focus on getting back on track. And remember, everything gets easier and easier with time and experience, and staying ideal-weighted is no exception! It is a new way to live, and that can take some adjustment time.

I no longer think of foods as "good" or "bad" relative to my weight. I really do eat whatever I want now. What has changed is what I want. I now want to feed my body fresh, whole foods, not processed items. One of my favourite meals is a big salad, with just about everything but the kitchen sink thrown in! I just love eating this way! I eat this way now because I truly enjoy it, not because I have to in order to manage my weight. I never, ever feel deprived. If I want something, I have it. I love desserts, especially anything with chocolate! I also just love good French fries, the kind with the potato skins still on them. I definitely like eating!

Although I ate meat until I was in my early 30s, I am a vegetarian now. What began 15 years ago as a month-long experiment to see what all the big deal about being veggie was quickly turned into my preferred choice. I just felt so much better not eating meat, especially red meat. However please don't think it was vegetarianism that caused my weight reduction, because it wasn't! Even as a veggie I have weighed as much as 235 pounds.

Even if you currently are a serious "fast-food junkie," please don't get all worked up and discouraged at the idea of (eventually) eating more healthfully. Take this journey one step at a time. You may never get to the stage where you love and appreciate a big salad and you may always want to eat a Big Mac! Please remember, your weight has very little to do with the actual food and so much more to do with the way you see yourself and where your autopilot is directing you. I am just sharing my choices with you; you are free to make your own!

I have really enjoyed sharing what I've learned with you. It has been very therapeutic for me too! At a recent pre-launch event of this book, after I spoke to the crowd, I was overwhelmed by how many people came up to me and made comments about how I was telling their life story. I felt a real sense of community, of belonging. When I began this book, I really had no idea if anyone was going to care to read it, and if they did, what they would think. I am so honoured that so many people are being touched by my story and are wanting to share with me their own weight journeys. I have actually been very surprised by how similar our stories are, and how I feel "lighter" both physically and emotionally as we all share and learn together. I have since wondered how differently my life might have turned out if I had a resource like *Why Are You Weighting?* early in my journey. I think I might not have felt the same isolation and desperation if I had known others were facing what I had been facing. So I encourage you to share this information with anyone you know who battles/battled their weight. Together we can accomplish great things as more and more people look in the mirror and ask themselves the question *Why Are You Weighting?*

To Your Success,

Stacey

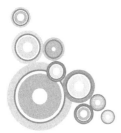

Recommended Resources

IN CHAPTER 8 OF *Why Are You Weighting?* I talked about sleep, water and nutrition and promised to let you know what I found as solutions for these challenges. Well, what I found was an innovative concept called The Wellness Home, developed by a 32-year-old Japanese wellness company called Nikken, now based out of California.

A Wellness Home helps to keep your body healthy and in balance, through attention to four different areas: Rest and Relaxation, Environment, Nutrition, and Fitness. However, as I mentioned in a previous chapter, no one likes to change, and this is where I think Nikken really fits in.

The Wellness Home concept does not require you to make any big changes to your lifestyle. You just keep doing what you've been doing, only now you do it using a Nikken technology instead of whatever you have been using. This will make more sense as you continue reading!

With regard to sleep, Nikken produces the Kenko Sleep System, which consists of three special components: a mattress (or mattress pad), a quilt, and a pillow. What these three components do is create a sleeping environment that just lets your body relax and sleep more effectively. Not only get to sleep, but also stay asleep! The Sleep System contains a number of patented technologies that actually help your body do what it is supposed to do while you are sleeping! It also supports your bones and muscles so that you are really comfortable during the night and when you wake up. There is special technology in the Sleep System to ensure that you are maintaining the right temperature as you sleep, regardless of whether you share your bed with a partner, or sleep alone.

In fact, this Sleep System is so effective that the World Federation of Chiropractic gave it an exclusive endorsement in 2005.

For me, using this Sleep System caused me to sleep. Really deep sleep. Restorative sleep. Healthy sleep. And boy did I feel differently during the day once I got going on this. My mood swings became a thing of the past, my caffeine addiction abated, and my weight fluctuated so much less! I became a happier, easier person to be with. My whole life was affected positively when I finally started sleeping!

So, if you are not sleeping, really sleeping, you need a solution. (Sleep medications are not a long-term solution.) And the solution I recommend is the personalized Nikken Sleep System. It just works. After all, you've got to sleep anyway. Why not sleep in the absolute best environment for your body? Simple solution to a big problem. You can learn more about this Sleep System at www.WhyAreYouWeighting.com and clicking on the Wellness Home link.

NOW, ON TO A DRINKING WATER SOLUTION.

TODAY WE HAVE myriad options with regard to drinking water: tap, reverse osmosis, distilled, filtered, or spring water. And believe it or not, any one of these can be what is found inside a "bottled water" container, including tap water.

If you think about nature, and what is supposed to happen in nature, you would realize that what we are drinking now is not what Mother Nature intended for us. In a perfect natural setting, you would have easy access to beautiful, fresh, delicious water that had just melted and run down from the snow-topped mountain after the sunlight had warmed it. This water would be filled with the healthy minerals that it would have picked up as it ran over all the rocks along the way down the side of the mountain. It would be energizing, clean, healthy and delicious, and your body would love it!

Well that's what Nikken has duplicated in their home drinking water systems. These systems not only strip the water clean of all the contaminants, but then they go a couple of steps further to produce mountain-quality spring water right out of your own tap! For literally pennies a litre/quart, you can incorporate the Nikken water system into your home, and then just watch what happens to the health and energy levels of those drinking it.

So again, a simple solution to the global problem of where is the clean drinking water going to come from. Doesn't get much easier or more convenient than from your own tap now does it? Please visit www.WhyAreYouWeighting.com to

learn more about the Nikken Water Sytems by clicking on the
Wellness Home link.

AND SO WHAT ABOUT NUTRITION?

MOST PEOPLE KNOW THERE is a problem with
drinking water quality, but few know that there is also a
problem with soil quality. And since most of our food is grown
either from the soil, or it feeds off something that is grown in
the soil, this is a big problem.

And I am not even talking about additives such as
pesticides. I am talking about the very constituents of the soil
itself. ("Organic" only means that no pesticides or chemicals
were used in the growing of the food; it doesn't mean that the
soil was remineralized prior to planting.)

The U.S. Government produced a paper called Document
264 in 1936, which stated that the American soils were grossly
depleted of all the basic minerals. And then in 1992, The Earth
Summit reported that soils the world over were all seriously
depleted of the basic minerals, anywhere from 55 to 85 percent
short of what they had contained 100 years prior.

If a plant doesn't get the proper minerals during the
growing stage, will not be able to produce the vitamins that are
supposed to be in it.

So what this means is that even if we are really diligent
about our diets, and eat only healthy food, we are still not
getting what our bodies need to be fully nourished.

The only way to fully ensure that the body is getting its required levels of vitamins and minerals is to supplement our diets.

The supplement industry is growing at a furious pace to meet consumer demand. Many companies are now in the supplement industry, some with good products, and some with not-so-good!

Once again, Nikken has made it simple and easy to get the nourishment your body requires through three basic nutritional products. The first is Jade Greenzymes, a powder made from organic baby barley grass that you just mix with water or fruit juice. This powder is like energy in a glass, and will help to feed your body right down to the cells!

The second product is a juice called Ciaga, which is a blend of 21 different fruit nectars and extracts. Just one ounce of this delicious juice offers your body all kinds of nutrition to keep you healthy. This wonder juice helps your heart and lungs, your digestive system, and your immune system, and, all in all, just makes a healthier, stronger you!

And then the third product is a daily vitamin and mineral packet, with specific formulas for men and for women, because our needs are different. These packets are called Kenzen Daily Wellness, and in addition to the vitamins and minerals, they also contain Omega-3 and -6 fatty acids, as well as digestive enzymes to ensure that your body can digest it all, and use it all!

Nikken will arrange it so that all your nutritional products can be delivered to your door, once a month, to make staying on track just so easy. No more running out and not having time to get to the store to pick up what you are missing. No more standing in the store, in front of a wall of supplements, wondering what you are supposed to be taking. No more taking supplements, that are simply not the quality your body requires...just simple, easy nourishment you take once a day. It doesn't get much easier than this! Please visit www.WhyAreYouWeighting.com to learn more about Nikken's Nutrionals, by clicking on the Wellness Home link.

And lastly, I just want to talk about a great pair of walking shoes that Nikken has invented, called the Cardiostrides. These shoes look just like typical sports shoes, but there is a big difference in what they are doing. The Cardiostrides have weighted insoles in them, which has two great advantages for your body. First, the extra weight causes your body to burn upto 25 percent more calories with every step you take. Now those of us who can walk do, so by wearing these shoes whenever you are walking, you are giving your weight reduction/maintenance an added boost. These shoes can be worn as part of a dedicated walking program, or they can just be used during your day-to-day routines, such as walking around the mall or grocery store, getting to the bus in the morning, as you do your vacuuming, etc. I wear these shoes whenever I have to walk anywhere, knowing that I am doing something extra good for my body!

The weight in the Cardiostrides also helps with any problems in the ankles, knees, hips, or lower back because the weight gently forces your body to walk more correctly. And the shoes work to tone your legs, your stomach, and your behind, so you not only feel better, you actually look better too! I encourage you to learn more about these shoes from Nikken at www.WhyAreYouWeighting.com and clicking on the Wellness Home link.

I really hope that you will take a look at the Nikken Wellness Home. It is an investment in your health that will pay off for years to come, and will ensure that your body is rested, properly hydrated, and meeting its basic nutritional requirements, which means that you won't be having uncontrollable cravings that cause you to break down in your resolve to permanently maintain your weight.

Please visit www.WhyAreYouWeighting.com to learn more about creating your own Wellness Home. Your body will thank you!

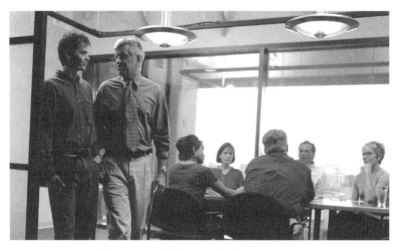

SHARE THIS MESSAGE

Bulk Discounts

Discounts start at a low number of copies, ranging from 30% to 50% off based on the quantity chosen.

Custom Publishing

Would you like a private label? or a customization to suit your needs. We could even highlight specific chapters.

Sponsorship

Would you like to sponsor this book? It's a great way to advertise your product or service in a unique way!

Dynamic Speakers

Authors are available to you, to share their expertise at your event!

*Call LifeSuccess Publishing at 1-800-473-7134 or email
info@lifesuccesspublishing.com for more information*